C0046 26706

D1424328

Toddler gym

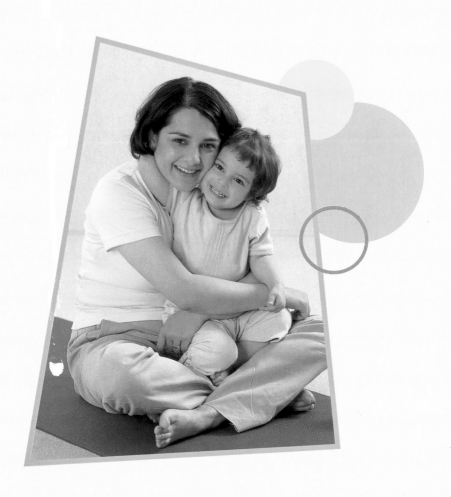

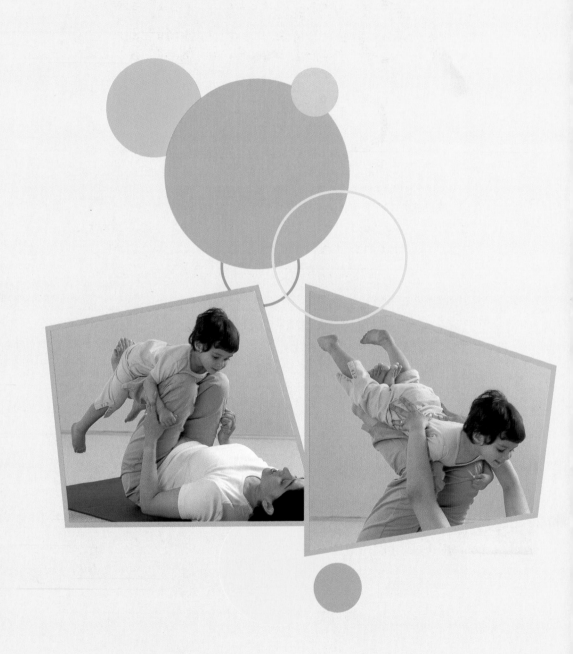

Toddler gym

Exercises, activities and games
to promote your child's movement, posture
and balancing skills

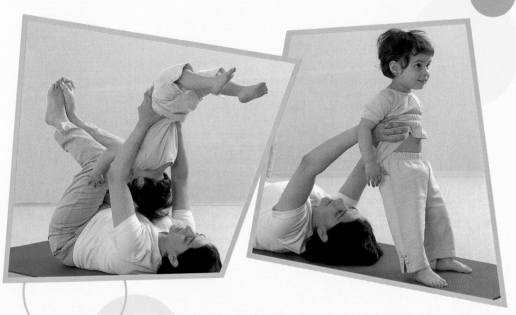

Peter Walker

CARROLL & BROWN PUBLISHERS LIMITED

Dedicated to
Chandana and Tai

This edition first published in 2006 in the United Kingdom by

Carroll & Brown Publishers Limited
20 Lonsdale Road
London NW6 6RD

Managing Editor Becky Alexander, Michelle Bernard
Art Editor Evie Loizides-Graham
Photographer Jules Selmes

Text © Peter Walker, 2002
Illustrations and compilation © Carroll & Brown Limited 2002

A CIP catalogue record for this book is available from the British Library.

ISBN 1-904760-28-7

10987654321

Previously published under the title
Hop, Skip & Jump

Glasgow City Council Cultural & Leisure Services Libraries Info. & Learning L		
C 004626706		
Askews		15-Dec-2010
613.710833 FH		£6.99

The mo ... of this
work h ... ns and

All right ... d in any
materi ... um by
electronic ... ome other
use of ... pyright
owner, e ... Designs
and P ... by the
Copyrigh ... VIP 9HE.
Applicati ... duce any
p. ... er.

Reproduced in Singapore by Colourscan
Printed and bound in Spain by Bookprint

Disclaimer: The author and publisher specifically disclaim any responsibility
for any liability, loss or risk (personal, financial or otherwise) that may be
claimed or incurred as a consequence – directly or indirectly – of the use
and/or application of any of the contents of this publication.

Contents

Introduction

Children love to move. Even when they are obliged to sit quietly, they will wiggle their toes and tap their feet and rock themselves backwards and forwards.

Making full use of a child's natural love of movement, this book presents a variety of soft gymnastic games and techniques to help to maintain suppleness and flexibility as your youngster gets bigger and stronger. These safe and fun games and exercises promote continued fitness during an important period of physical development.

From birth onwards, babies stretch their limbs and twist and bend their bodies to create a wonderful range of movement and establish the flexibility of the body's major joints. Over the first 12 months or so, they develop the motor skills necessary for independence.

Having first established flexibility, toddlers go on to develop strength, mainly by lifting and carrying their rapidly increasing body weight. Unless children continue to

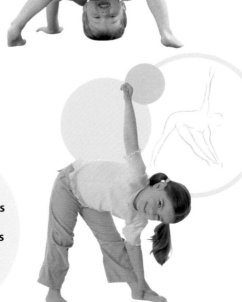

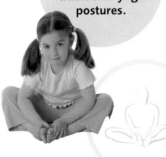

A number of the stretches shown here are based on traditional yoga postures.

These are ideally suited to children, since many yoga postures are actually based upon positions and movements naturally made by the developing child.

experience a wide variety and range of movement once they are on their feet, like all weightlifters they will begin to lose some of their inborn flexibility. So it's at this stage that some work has to be done to maintain their natural suppleness.

This book will help you to ensure the health and fitness of all the major muscles and joints and show you how to help your children retain their flexibility, increasing their ability to effectively perform a wide range of movement as they grow older and more adventurous.

The benefits of soft gymnastics are not only physical. A child who moves freely and gracefully is self-confident and relaxed.

And, in practising the games and exercises presented in this book, you and your children will work cooperatively. As your children rely on your guiding hands to try new postures and shapes with their bodies, you will encourage greater trust in your relationship. With each gentle stretch, your children will grow increasingly comfortable in their bodies – steadier on their feet and more certain in their responses.

But the ultimate aim of this book is pleasure. It has been created to ensure you have fun with your children. Give yourself up to the spirit of the child – in that way, the time you spend together will be enjoyable, full of laughter and fun and love.

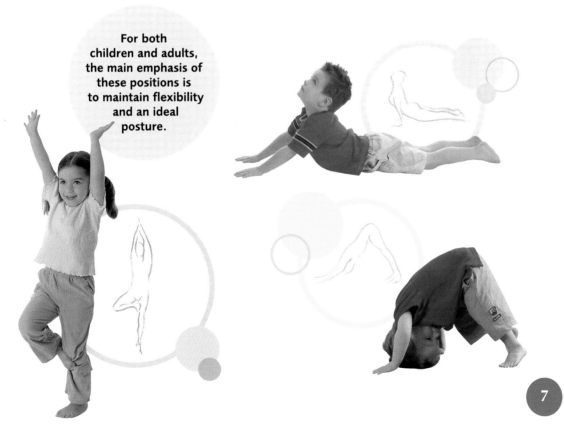

For both children and adults, the main emphasis of these positions is to maintain flexibility and an ideal posture.

Developmental Milestones

From birth to around three years of age, your child develops new motor skills with astounding speed. It's amazing to watch the transformation that occurs over such a short span of time, as your child grows from being a helpless infant, totally dependent on carers to satisfy every need and desire, into a strong and independent toddler, able to hold his own, even away from the home.

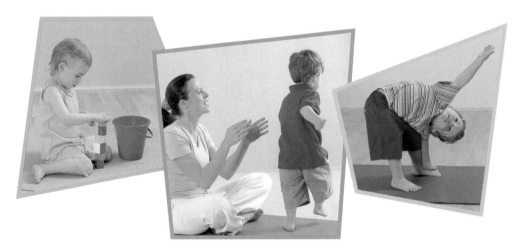

All children everywhere follow a well-documented sequence of developmental stages, but the age at which an individual child reaches each stage varies greatly. There are usually differences in individual patterns; some children, for example, spend a lot more time crawling than others. While it is helpful to be aware of developmental milestones, so you can help to promote the skills your child is working towards, it is important not to judge your child, or compare his abilities to any other children of the same age, except in the most general terms. However, if you are concerned that your child appears very late in developing any motor skills, you should consult your GP or health visitor for advice.

Infancy

During the first 15 to 18 months, a baby must adjust from the weightless environment of his mother's womb to learning to hold himself up against the force of gravity, the strongest force on earth. During this time, he will develop many motor and tactile skills that will start him on the road to independence. Broadly, a baby will develop flexibility following a distinct pattern. First, he will open the front of his body, moving from a foetal position to stretching the muscles in the front while straightening and strengthening his back, and flexing and encouraging his body's many joints to move.

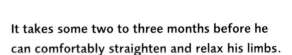

It takes some two to three months before he can comfortably straighten and relax his limbs.

At 3 MONTHS he will have a degree of head control and, lying on his tummy, he will have enough strength in his spine to be able to lift his head and shoulders from the floor, bearing his weight on his forearms. By the end of the sixth month, he will have full head control.

At 9 MONTHS, a baby will probably be able to sit upright unsupported. When lying on the floor he will start to roll around, getting his first experience of freedom of movement. This is when he may begin to crawl and to stand, pulling himself up on furniture or other supports.

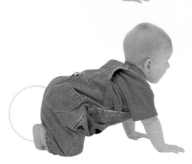

9

The toddler years

Once on the move, a child is like a little weightlifter. By lifting and carrying his ever-increasing bodyweight, he will strengthen rapidly. Like any weightlifter, however, unless he continues to make a full range of bodily movement, his muscles and joints will begin to tighten and his body will become less flexible. This is why it is important to allow your developing child time to move freely, rather than confining him for long periods to playpens or walkers.

13 MONTHS is about the average age at which a child will learn to walk unaided. At this age he is often able to crawl upstairs.

At 15 MONTHS, a toddler can move from sitting to standing without support and can kneel unaided to collect objects from the floor. He can push large, wheeled toys on level ground. He can probably seat himself in a chair by climbing up on it, then turning around to sit.

At 18 MONTHS, a toddler can walk backwards and forwards, run, pull and push toys, and throw a ball without toppling over.

By 21 MONTHS, he can lean forwards from standing to pick up objects from the floor without falling, and he can also squat comfortably.

At TWO YEARS, a toddler can run, safely avoiding obstacles, squat to rest and play and then stand easily. He can kick a ball without falling over. He can walk up and downstairs, placing two feet on each step and holding a handrail, and he can sit astride and propel large, wheeled toys.

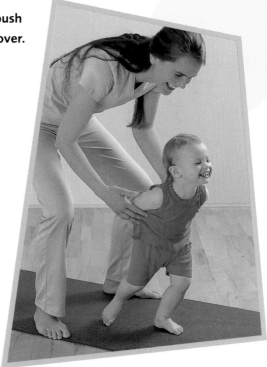

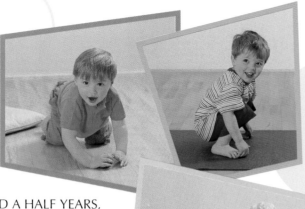

At TWO AND A HALF YEARS, a child can jump with both feet together and stand and walk on tiptoe. He can walk upstairs unaided, one foot at a time, although when he goes downstairs, he will still place two feet on each step and hold a handrail. He will now be very active and will walk, run and jump freely, at the same time as he still crawls, rolls, sits, kneels and squats on the floor.

At THREE YEARS, a child can stand briefly on one leg, climb with agility and turn corners and avoid obstacles while pushing large mobile toys.

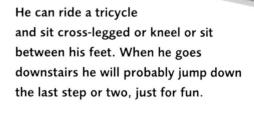

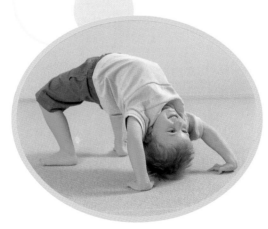

He can ride a tricycle and sit cross-legged or kneel or sit between his feet. When he goes downstairs he will probably jump down the last step or two, just for fun.

Between THREE AND FOUR YEARS of age, many mobile skills are perfected. Your child will become bolder and more confident, ready to venture into the world with increasing independence.

11

Do's and Don't s of Soft Gymnastics

Do

Practise soft gymnastics only when both you and your child are in the mood. Your child will sense any tension or reluctance that you feel.

Keep it fun. Talk and sing, and fully engage your child while you practise these exercises together.

Set up a soft, non-slip surface on which to exercise. Put pillows around your practice area to cushion any falls and to provide a cosy area for relaxing cuddles when you finish.

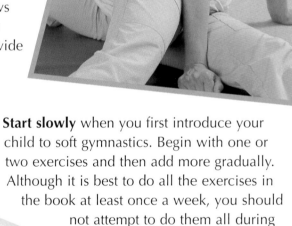

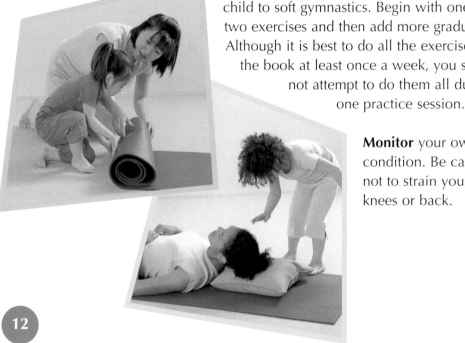

Start slowly when you first introduce your child to soft gymnastics. Begin with one or two exercises and then add more gradually. Although it is best to do all the exercises in the book at least once a week, you should not attempt to do them all during one practice session.

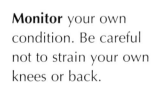

Monitor your own condition. Be careful not to strain your own knees or back.

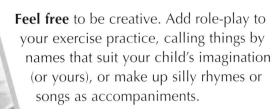

Feel free to be creative. Add role-play to your exercise practice, calling things by names that suit your child's imagination (or yours), or make up silly rhymes or songs as accompaniments.

Stop before your child gets bored. It's always better to leave your child wanting more.

Don't

DON'T perform these or any other flexibility exercises with your child if she is hypermobile, or 'floppy'.

DON'T practise soft gymnastics if your child is unwell, has any swelling or bruising or if she complains of pain. In this event, consult your physician immediately.

DON'T try to do too many of the exercises at any one time, unless you are enjoying yourself and your child insists on continuing. As you both gain confidence, your soft gymnastics sessions will naturally get longer.

DON'T do any of these exercises against the will of your child. If she is unwilling or unenthusiastic, you will only increase your child's resistance. Remember that this is something you do *with* your child, not *to* your child.

DON'T use force to move your child into any position. These exercises may well reveal areas of stiffness in your child, which may be overcome with regular, gentle practice, carefully following the guidelines in each exercise.

SPINE, CHEST AND SHOULDERS

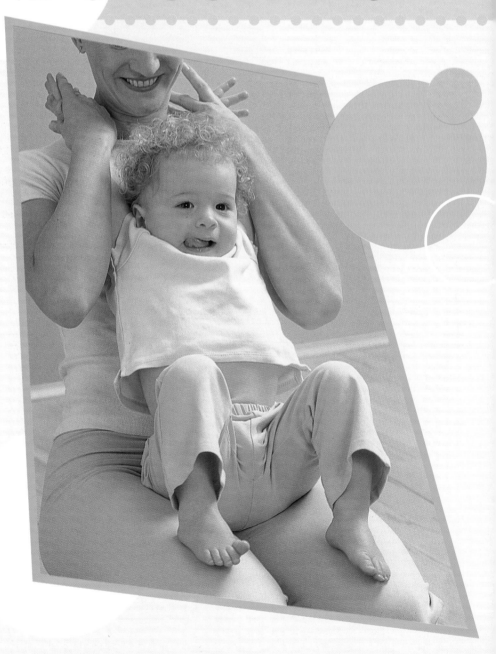

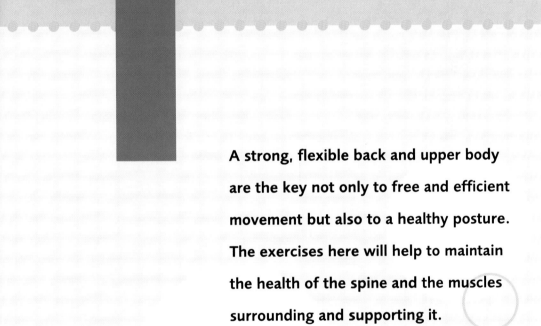

**A strong, flexible back and upper body
are the key not only to free and efficient
movement but also to a healthy posture.
The exercises here will help to maintain
the health of the spine and the muscles
surrounding and supporting it.**

Clap and Shake

If you start when your child is quite young, you can encourage him to develop his upper body flexibility. As soon as your baby is able to comfortably lift his arms upwards, you can begin to help him to 'loosen up'.

This stretch is beneficial for babies as they begin to mobilise their arms, but you also can continue to practise these gentle moves with your toddler in a variety of different situations. Working together to stretch his arms out and up will help him to open his chest and gently warm up his spine before he tries some of the more vigorous stretches later in the book. It can also help him to relax, not only at the end of a playful exercise session, but at other times of the day as well.

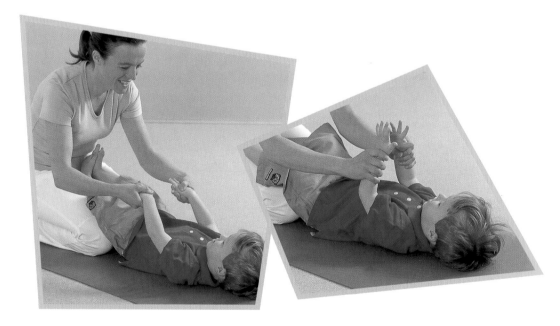

1 Sit comfortably on a cushion, with your child lying on his back facing you. Taking his hands, give his arms a little shake before bringing them towards his body.

2 Gently shake both arms before clapping his hands together. Now open his arms in line with his shoulders. Repeat a few times, keeping your movements light.

Practice Point

Do not force your child's arms in any way. If he resists raising his arms, hold his elbows and tap his arms quickly but gently against the floor, without straightening them.

3 Take his elbows and tap his arms gently but quickly against the floor a few times to completely relax both arms from the shoulders.

4 Shake your child's arms gently, then lift them over his head. You can punctuate this with lots of kisses on his chest, just for fun.

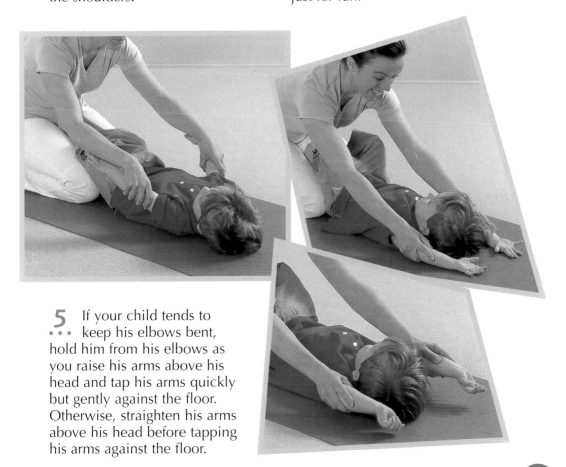

5 If your child tends to keep his elbows bent, hold him from his elbows as you raise his arms above his head and tap his arms quickly but gently against the floor. Otherwise, straighten his arms above his head before tapping his arms against the floor.

Circle Massage

As important to posture as it is to breathing, this exercise opens and relaxes the chest and shoulders from end to end and top to bottom, and also closes and strengthens the back muscles in the same way.

This stretch may be particularly useful when you want to help your child to calm down, as it promotes relaxation. As you lift your child's arms upwards in line with her head, her shoulder blades drop back and down, fully opening her chest and relaxing her shoulders. This should induce a delicious feeling of serenity that pervades the upper chest and shoulders. Your child's breathing will slow down and deepen, inducing a relaxed and calm state.

As your growing child spends more time standing and sitting, it is important to lay the groundwork for good posture in the future. The spine is only as good as the muscles that support it, so strengthening the muscles that support the spine is an important step on the road to a healthy posture.

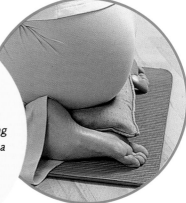

Practice Point

Make sure you are sitting comfortably, because any discomfort you may feel can be transferred to your child. If kneeling on the floor is difficult, try placing a cushion between your feet and your buttocks, or under your buttocks.

1 Sit comfortably on the floor with your child on your lap.

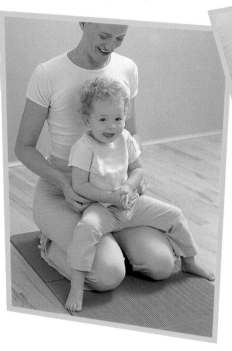

2 Once you are both settled, bring your hands onto her chest and, using the palms of your hands, massage her chest and shoulders with a few light, circular movements.

3 Give her arms a gentle shake, then open them out sideways. Massage her arms by gently pulling them through your hands, from her shoulder to forearm, 3 or 4 times.

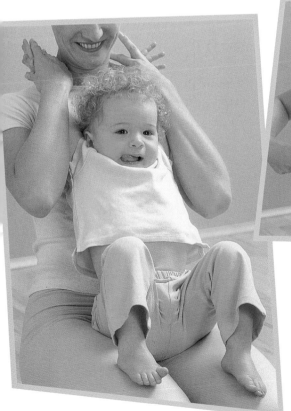

4 Lean back, shake her arms gently, and lift them above her head in line with her ears. Rock gently from side to side, and give her arms another gentle shake to finish.

Sideways Rock

Today, with the emphasis on putting babies on their backs to sleep and play, some toddlers may have missed out on valuable tummy time in the earlier stages of their physical development. The development of a strong back begins in infancy, as your baby raises herself up from the floor when she is lying on her tummy.

The following exercise is a good remedy for a child who may not have had much tummy time. But any child will benefit from being encouraged to open and relax her chest and tummy, strengthening her back as she does so.

It is also a good first step for young children who are a little reluctant to arch their backs or open their chests. If your child feels vulnerable when she stretches the front of her body, this is a gentle introduction to the movement. As she gently arches her back, supported by your legs and very near to your comforting arms, her confidence will grow.

Practice Point

Pay attention to your child's head and neck; her neck should be aligned with her spine. If she begins to strain her head upwards, help her back to a sitting position.

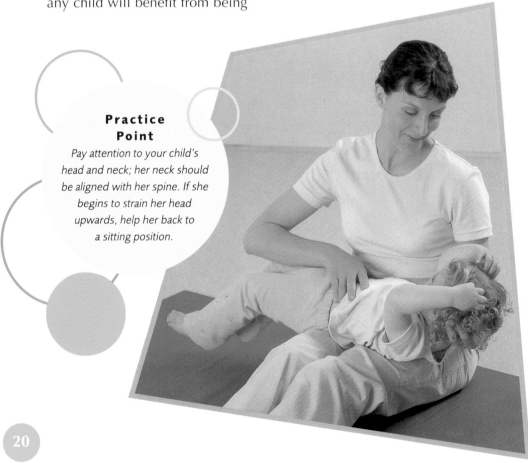

1. Sit comfortably on the floor or on a cushion with slightly bent knees. Let your child sit sideways over your thighs, and support the back of her head with one hand and both legs with the other as she begins to relax back over your legs.

2. Shake her legs gently as you lower them, letting her arch backwards over your thighs. If your child begins to lift her head, or if she expresses any discomfort, help her to lift herself upright again.

3. Shake her arms gently and lift them above her head in line with her ears. While her hands rest on the floor, rock her gently from side to side. Give her arms another gentle shake before bringing her upright.

Rub Your Tummy

When small children first sit and stand, they naturally maintain a beautifully straight back. A strong, healthy spine is necessary for this ideal posture, which benefits the body's total structure.

A strong spine and good posture also conserve energy: when the spine is straight, the body's weight is distributed evenly downwards through its joints, but if a child slumps, rounding her spine and hollowing her chest, the weight can no longer be supported by balanced bones, and extra muscular effort is required.

You can help your child to maintain the integrity of her spinal column throughout childhood and beyond

by practising gentle backbends together. These stretches strengthen the spine and also maintain its flexibility and range of motion.

Offering your child a light massage, through stroking and gentle percussion, will enhance the positive effects of the backbend, because it will encourage total relaxation of the chest and tummy while the muscles are stretching.

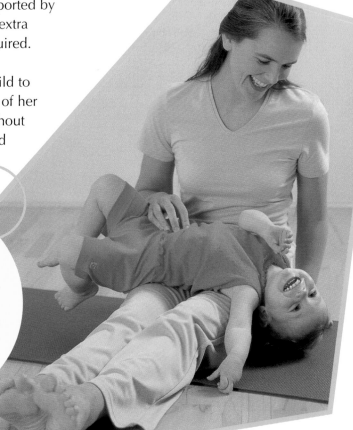

Practice Point

If your child is uncomfortable doing backbends, you can talk or sing to her to help her to relax. Proceed slowly, stopping if she is too reluctant, and offer love and reassurance.

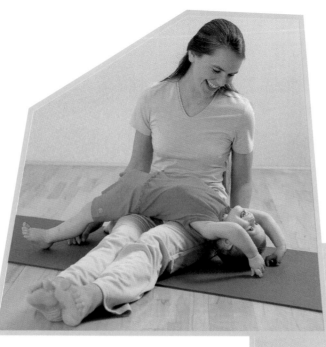

1 Begin with your child in the gentle backbend over your legs described in Sideways Rock (see page 20).

2 Using the relaxed weight of your hand, stroke your child's tummy in a clockwise direction, continuing with gentle strokes down her thighs. If your child resists and wants to lift her head or feet, help her to sit up again.

3 Cup your hands together, and lightly and rhythmically pat her chest.

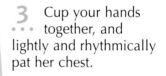

Bounce and Roll

This backbend is specially designed to preserve and improve the strength and flexibility of your child's back. While it is immensely therapeutic, the exercise should also be a source of pleasure. Not only will the exercise benefit your child's physicality, but it's also an entertaining way for you and your child to spend time together. If you place the emphasis on having fun, your youngster will enjoy the experience – and so will you.

An exercise ball can add extra fun and interest. Children naturally respond to balls and love to play with them.

Let your child fool around with the ball as he chooses, because free play is also extremely valuable for your child's physical, creative and emotional development.

Bouncing your child gently while he stretches takes the focus away from the exercise itself and makes the activity a playful one. Your child will not feel any pressure towards achievement but will be able to enjoy the movement and the stretch. You can engage your child in the moment by maintaining eye contact and singing or talking together while he is on the ball. This will also help to reassure him if he is uncertain about the position.

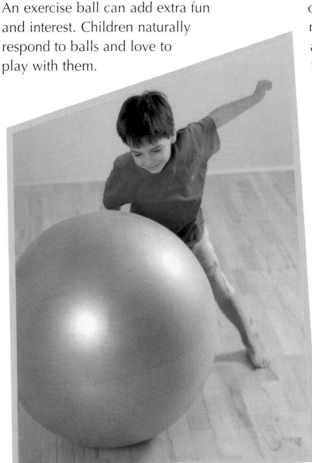

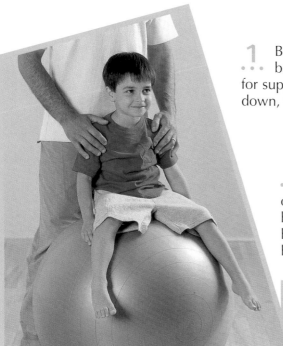

1 Begin by sitting your child on the ball, holding him by the shoulders for support. Gently bounce him up and down, to help him get used to the ball.

2 When he is comfortable, encourage him to lie backwards over the ball. Once he has relaxed his head and legs, hold him from his hip and opposite shoulder and roll him gently backwards and forwards.

3 Bring him back to the top of the ball and change your grip to hold him from both sides of his hips, gently bouncing him up and down a few times.

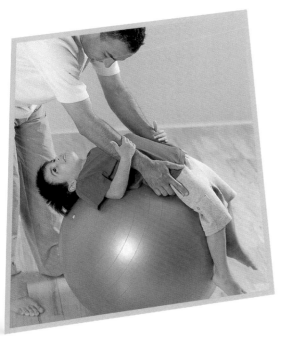

Using an exercise ball

When you work with your child on an exercise ball, remember that it is unstable. Always make sure that your child is on the centre of the ball so that he does not roll sideways or backwards without your support. At first, as you both get used to working with the ball, it may be helpful to keep the ball slightly deflated so that it is a little more stable.

25

Rolling on the Ball

The abdomen is known as the centre of tranquillity. If you place your hand upon your child's tummy when he is relaxed and happy, it will feel as soft and malleable as a marshmallow. Alternatively, if you place your hand across his tummy when he is upset or unhappy, it will feel as hard as a rock. Helping your child maintain a relaxed tummy is of great benefit to his future health and well-being. Whatever we are doing, our performance is improved if we maintain abdominal relaxation, because when the abdomen is tense, our concentration is impeded by the sensations of inner discomfort. In addition, holding on to the muscles in this way is tiring, depleting the body's energy.

The stretch demonstrated here not only relaxes the abdomen but aids digestion. As the abdominal muscles relax, the stretch relieves excessive wind and creates space for the abdominal organs to function more efficiently. This exercise is a continuation of the Bounce and Roll (see page 24).

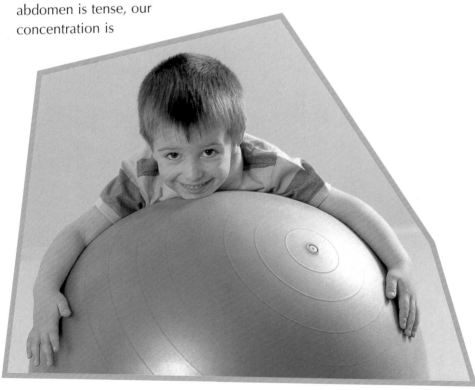

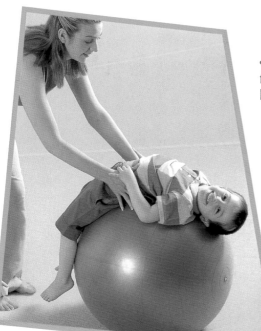

1 Place your child on his back on the ball. Hold him from the hips, and encourage him to relax back over the ball.

2 Bring him slowly back to a standing position with his feet touching the floor and his head and spine remaining comfortably arched backwards over the ball.

3 Keeping hold of his hips, roll your child slowly backwards and forwards, encouraging him to lie back over the top of the ball again, this time with his arms stretched out sideways.

Practice Point

Suggest that your child imagine that he is a part of the ball, and that he is sinking into the ball, as you bounce him gently. This can help a child to relax into the movement.

Advanced Rolling on the Ball

Movement is the most obvious sign of life, and the more fluidly the body moves, the more alive it appears. This is why observing – and sharing in – the joyous physical freedom of children is so invigorating.

The body's joints are crucial to free and spirited movement. Healthy joints are able to complete the full range of motion for which they are designed. Nowhere else in the body is this more important than in the spine, which supports and protects the body's central nervous system. A flexible spine ensures the healthy functioning of the nervous system and the free distribution of nerve impulses throughout the body.

Backbends such as this serve more than one purpose: they mobilise and strengthen the back at the same time as they stretch the front of the body.

As your child grows more experienced with backbends, you can gradually encourage her to take the stretch a bit further.

Here, in this more advanced variation on the previous exercise, she raises her arms over her head, creating a stretch that lengthens the body from fingertips to toes, with the ball supporting her safely.

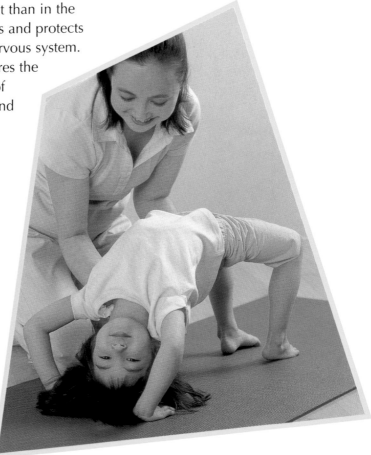

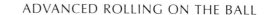

1 As your child lies across the top of the ball, hold her firmly from the hips. Once she feels comfortable and secure, bounce and roll her gently backwards and forwards, keeping her close to the top of the ball.

2 Change your grip to hold her firmly from her knees and ask her to stretch her arms back over her head. Bounce her, and roll her further backwards. Ensure she keeps her head and neck relaxed.

3 Change your grip again, this time holding your child firmly by her ankles. Gently bounce and roll her further backwards, with her arms stretched over her head and her head and neck relaxed, until her hands touch or nearly touch the floor.

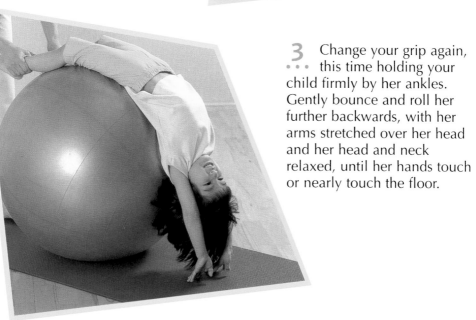

Supported Backbend

Working closely together with your child is an enormously satisfying experience. In this variation on the backbend, you use your own body to support your child, rather than relying on the ball. It is a simple and relaxing stretch for both you and your child.

As your child allows you to support his body weight, he is trusting in your ability to hold him safely. This kind of trust is the basis for some of the soft gymnastic games illustrated later in the book – and is also the basis for a fulfilling parent-child relationship.

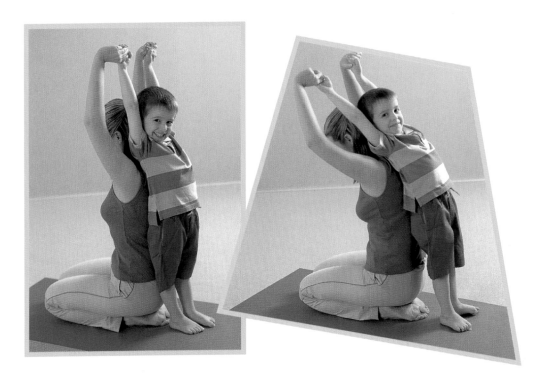

1 ••• As you sit comfortably on your feet, ask your child to stand with his back to yours. When you are both ready, have him lift his arms, and holding him firmly from his hands, give him a gentle shake to loosen and relax him before you begin.

2 ••• Making sure that your child remains comfortably relaxed, with the back of his head and upper back resting firmly against yours, lean forward slowly and take his weight. You should feel his head, upper and lower back and legs against your back.

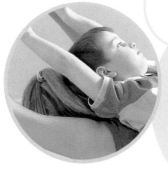

Practice Point

Throughout this exercise, it is important that you both keep your head and neck relaxed to avoid any strain on the back. If your child starts to raise his head, ask him to relax it back again.

3 Once your child is balanced upon your back with his feet off the floor, take great care not to lean too far forwards. Release his arms one at a time and transfer your grip to his hips. Holding him firmly, rock gently from side to side.

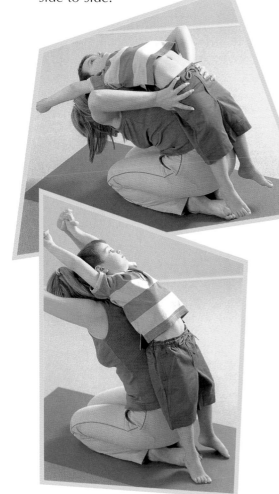

4 Still taking great care not to lean too far forwards and holding your child firmly from the hips, slowly raise up onto your knees and rock from side to side.

5 Carefully come back to a kneeling position, then slowly straighten your back until he is standing.

Standing Backbend

Oxygen is our first 'food of life'. We can go for weeks without food and days without water, but only minutes without oxygen.

Wholesome, deep breathing involves the interaction of many muscles, and the stretch shown here will help to keep them all functioning healthily.

When all the muscles involved in breathing function at their best, they achieve a rhythm known as abdominal breathing. This is more efficient than the rapid, shallow breathing that takes place if you only breathe from the chest. Abdominal breathing is also more relaxing. Shallow breathing is associated with feelings of anxiety and keeps the body in a constant state of alert, while long, slow, deep breaths are calming.

As you stretch together, observe your child's breathing rhythm. If he is breathing rapidly, soothe him and encourage him to take longer, deeper breaths.

Practice Point

If your child is initially a little reluctant to try this elevated backbend, let him get used to being lifted off the ground in this way by trying the same action as he lies on his front rather than his back.

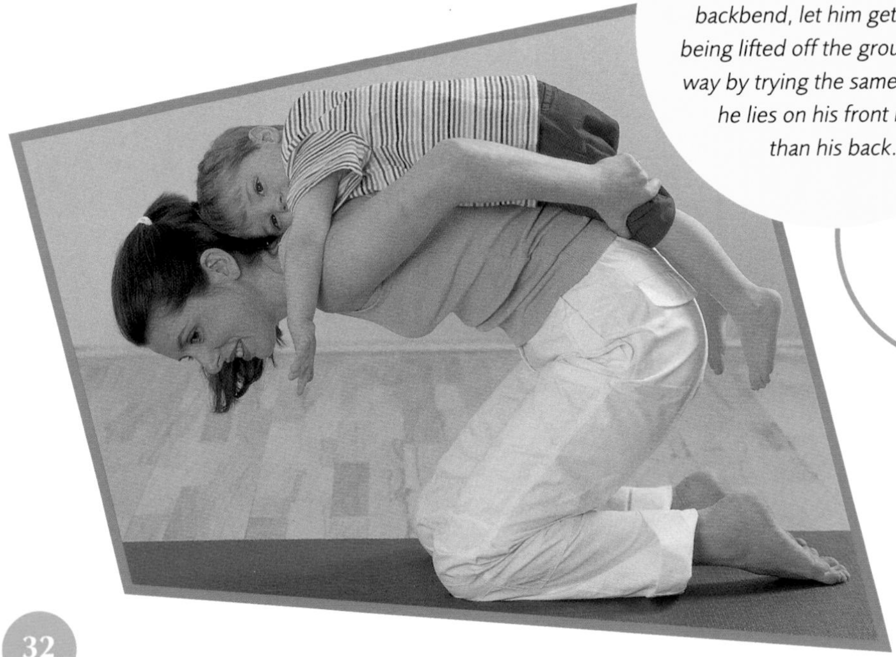

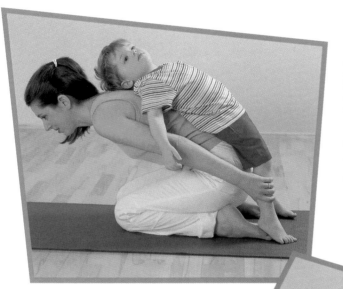

1 Kneel down on a cushion, with your buttocks resting on your heels, and ask your child to stand behind you, resting his back against yours. As you hold him from the lower legs, encourage him to relax against you and open his arms sideways. Rock gently from side to side.

2 Change your grip and hold him just above his ankles. Lean forwards and encourage your child to relax into this backbend over your back, extending his arms above his head. Make sure that his head is relaxed back against you, and that he is not straining his neck. Rock gently in this position.

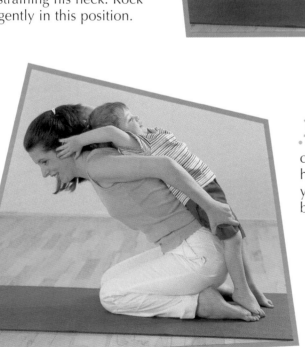

3 As you slowly start to straighten up again, change your grip to hold him from his hips, and as you sit up, gently bring him back to standing.

HIP AND LEG MOBILITY

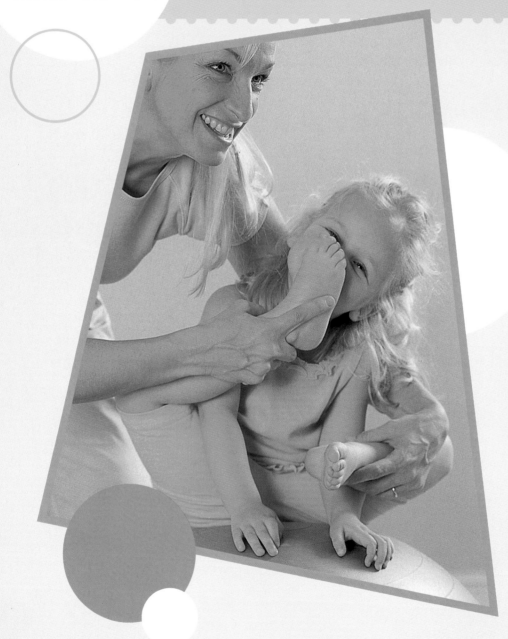

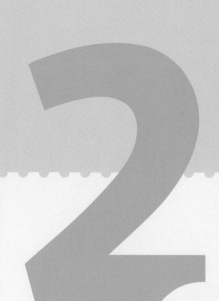

As your toddler launches herself wholeheartedly into new physical activities, she will rely on strong, agile legs to carry her. By performing exercises in this chapter, you will help to maintain the flexibility of her legs and hips.

Bicycle Claps

The hips and legs are the powerhouses of the body. They provide a sturdy base for sitting and standing, and are also the force for locomotion – first crawling, then walking, running, climbing, cycling and so on.

During the first months of life, a baby keeps his legs bent most of the time, and it is usually three to four months before he can fully relax his legs and let them remain completely extended.

As children grow, it is particularly important to maintain the flexibility of the legs. All activities involving the legs, such as running, or riding a scooter or a bicycle, are best performed with free joints.

1   Sit comfortably back on your feet, with your child lying on the floor on his back, with his feet pointing towards you.

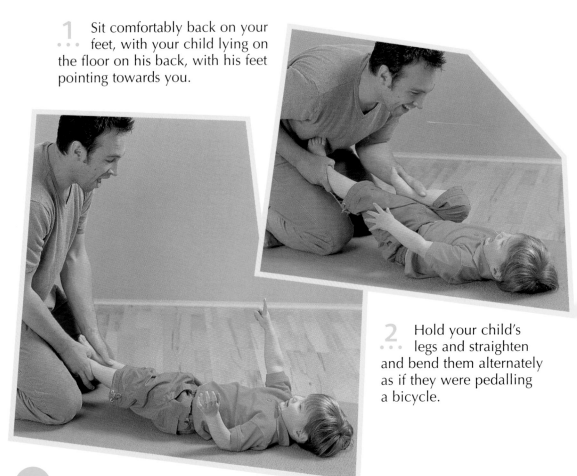

2   Hold your child's legs and straighten and bend them alternately as if they were pedalling a bicycle.

But because these movements are repetitive, they may tighten the muscles as they strengthen them and, over time, limit the range of movement by the joints. Over a long period, this can increase the wear and tear on active joints, making them more prone to injury.

Practising soft gymnastics is an ideal counterpoint to these repetitive activities. By enjoying exercises that lengthen the muscles and move the joints through their full range of motion, there is less chance of stiffness and consequently less chance of injury.

3 Now grasp your child's ankles and clap both feet together to relax the legs even further.

4 Gently press both feet towards his tummy and gently rock your child from side to side.

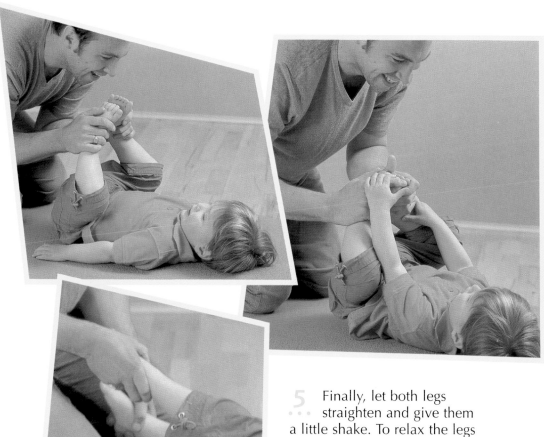

5 Finally, let both legs straighten and give them a little shake. To relax the legs further, pull them gently towards you a few times.

Kiss Your Toes

As toddlers become confident walkers, their legs gradually strengthen and they lose that early bow-legged 'cowboy' look. This straightening occurs as the inner thigh muscles contract, drawing the knees in to align with the hips. While this is essential for the hip joints to function efficiently, and for greater stability in standing and walking, it also means that the legs lose a measure of their flexibility.

Exercises like this one will help your growing child to retain the maximum amount of flexibility, without compromising the strength and stability she will require for an active and energetic life.

Here, you will help your child to draw her legs up towards her face. Young babies can do this without strain, sometimes even sucking their own toes for the sheer pleasure of it. Older children will find this stretch more of a challenge. Do not push the stretch: as soon as you feel any tension, allow your child's legs to relax down. But if your toddler can reach her toes to her mouth, the idea of sucking them is bound to elicit a giggle.

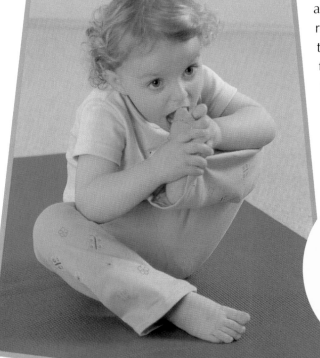

Fun and Games

As she practises this stretch, your child can pretend that her leg is a doll or a puppy that she is cradling and kissing.

1 ... Sit comfortably on the floor, with your child between your legs, leaning against you for support. Help her to cradle one shin in her arms, leaving her other leg relaxed and bent. Rock the raised leg gently side to side.

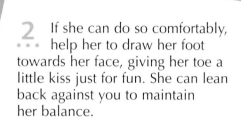

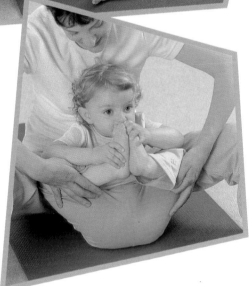

2 ... If she can do so comfortably, help her to draw her foot towards her face, giving her toe a little kiss just for fun. She can lean back against you to maintain her balance.

Alternatively

If your child has very flexible hips, she can try to move one foot at a time towards her face while she keeps her other leg extended straight out in front of her. This is a quite challenging variation, so should only be attempted once she is feeling very confident with the basic stretch.

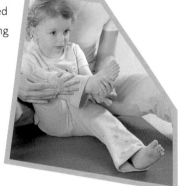

3 ... Let her raise both feet towards her face to give them both little kisses, as you support her lightly from the thighs.

Hip Openers

As your child becomes more physically active, her coordination will constantly improve, allowing her to engage in more varied and challenging activities. All the exercises in this book can help your child to further develop her coordination, but it is important to talk through the exercise as you work together. In this way you'll engage your child's mind as well as her body, and this mind-body connection is essential for motor coordination. Very young children will find the sound of your voice comforting, toddlers will learn the names of their body parts, and older children will gain some practice in following simple instructions.

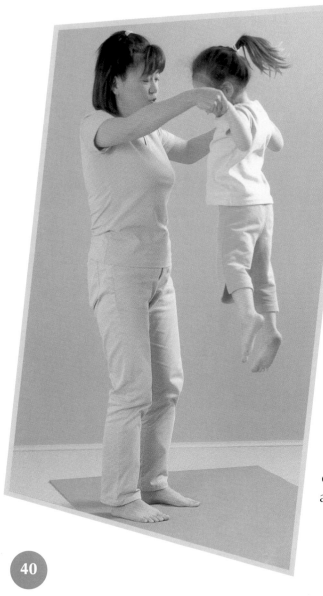

Soon enough, your child may try to turn the tables and instruct you in how to perform a stretch. Allowing your child to take the lead from time to time will greatly benefit her self-confidence.

By smoothly alternating the legs, this exercise will help to refine coordination. At the same time it continues to develop hip and leg flexibility, helping to relax the muscles that allow the legs to rotate open at the hips. It also adds a gentle stretch for the back.

1. Sit comfortably on the floor with your child lying down in front of you. Holding both of your child's feet, draw them towards her tummy, allowing her knees to bend and her legs to turn out at her hips.

2. Release the left foot. Pushing gently on the thigh of her right foot, take that foot towards her face, leaving the left leg bent and relaxed. Repeat on the other side.

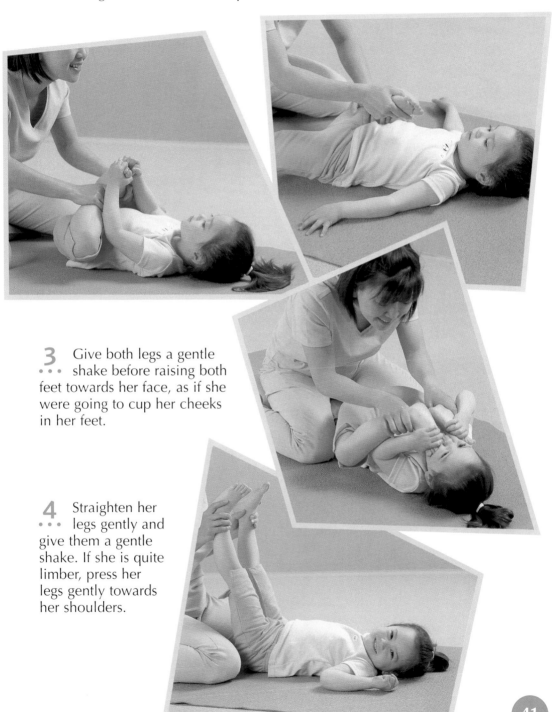

3. Give both legs a gentle shake before raising both feet towards her face, as if she were going to cup her cheeks in her feet.

4. Straighten her legs gently and give them a gentle shake. If she is quite limber, press her legs gently towards her shoulders.

Tailor Pose

The tailor pose – with the feet together and the knees open – mimics your child's first sitting posture. This is one of the healthiest ways to sit: from this secure base, the back remains straight, yet your child is free to lean forwards or sideways if he needs to. Sitting tailor style depends upon the flexibility of the hip joints, and in fact, as a child moves around in this position, perhaps leaning to pick up a toy or a book, he is effectively stretching his hip joints, ensuring their soundness. The more flexible the hips, the wider the base of the body and the more secure this makes sitting.

At first, as they learn to sit upright, most babies fall forwards or forwards and sideways. This is because they have not learned how to 'ground' themselves. All upright structures need good foundations, and once your child has learned how to push down on the base of his spine, sitting upright becomes easier. The following exercises, using the tailor pose and variations on it, will help relax your child's legs and keep his hip joints flexible, creating a secure foundation for a strong back.

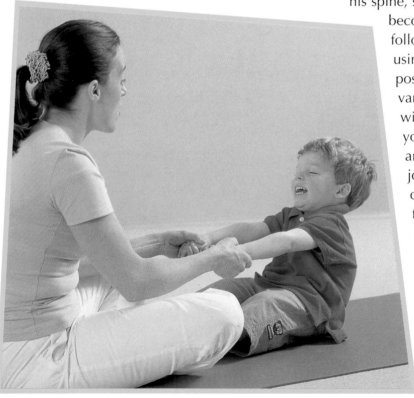

1 Sit comfortably on the floor with your child sitting on your lap facing outwards, his legs bent. Bring your arms under your child's arms and your hands over his ankles.

2 Gently bring your child's feet together, with his knees open, and rock him gently from side to side.

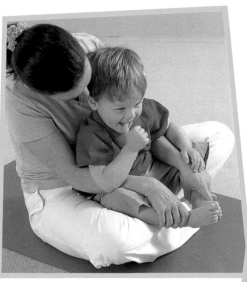

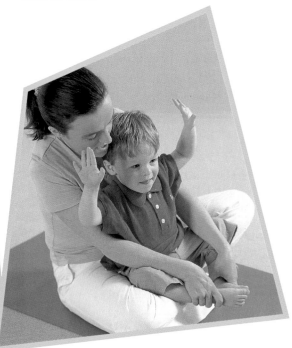

3 Let your child lean forwards some 45 degrees, supporting him firmly, and continue to rock him gently from side to side.

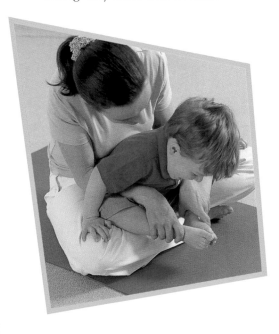

Learning to sit

Most babies are able to sit independently from about the age of five or six months. An infant continues to refine his sitting skills, first sitting supported by both arms, then sitting without arm support, then turning and reaching out as he sits. Eventually he will adopt a sitting position in which he sits back between his feet.

Many children continue to sit between their feet for several years. If your child does, try to make sure that his feet are turned inwards. If the feet are turned outwards in this position, the hip joints are more prone to dislocation.

Tailor Pose Swing

The flexibility of the ankles, knees and hips is vital to balanced posture and the free movement of the rest of the body. As children run, jump, leap, skip and cavort, they rely on the healthy functioning of their major joints to protect them from injury.

The ankle is a flexible arch that is 'sprung' to cushion the entire weight of the body. It can turn and rotate to adapt to uneven surfaces, allowing the body to remain upright when walking or running over uneven ground. The knees, the largest single joints in the body, are also able to bend and rotate inwards and outwards. The flexibility of the hip joints is vital to the integrity of the spine, because it allows the spine to remain straight when the body bends forward.

Because it involves all the key joints of the lower body, the tailor pose is an extremely beneficial stretch. This variation is one to practise with smaller children. They will delight in being swung around. Older children are better suited to practising tailor pose using the ball (see page 46).

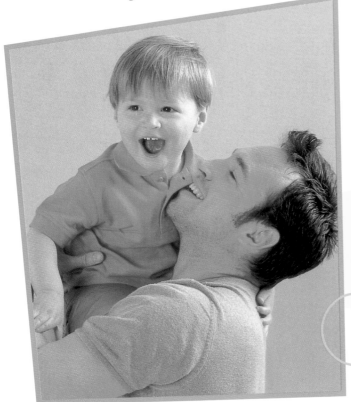

Practice Point
While you are swinging your child, be aware of your own back and shoulders, making sure that you do not strain yourself in any way.

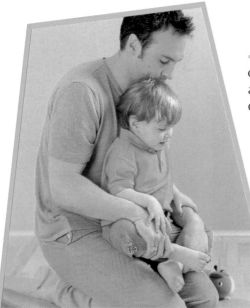

1 ••• Begin by sitting comfortably on your heels, with your child sitting on your lap, facing outwards. Bring your arms under his arms and your hands over his ankles.

2 ••• Push the soles of his feet together, allowing his knees to open outwards, and let him lean forwards around 45 degrees as you support his abdomen with your forearms.

3 ••• Holding your child securely in this position, raise yourself up on your knees. With your shoulders relaxed, swing him gently from side to side as he continues to lean forwards.

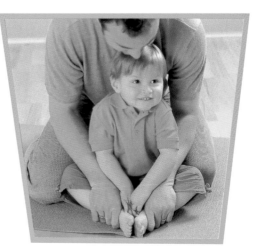

4 ••• Kneel back down before lowering your child gently into your lap. Finish with hugs and kisses.

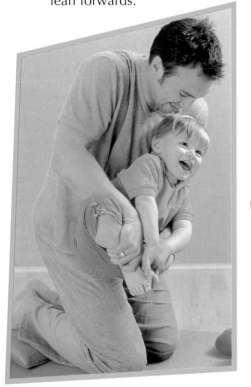

Tailor Pose Ball Practice

Once children begin to attend play groups, nurseries or pre-schools, they often will need to sit 'cross-legged' on the floor for a variety of activities. Cross-legged sitting is a variation of the tailor pose, and these exercises will ensure your child's comfort as she moves out into the world. Being able to sit comfortably will help her to maintain her concentration on whatever activity is taking place.

Even at home, it is a good idea to encourage your child to sit on the floor rather than on easy chairs or sofas. On the floor, a young child will unconsciously adopt a healthy posture, with a straight, balanced spine, while sitting on a soft chair or sofa will lead to your child curving her spine and jutting her chin forwards.

Many adults owe their poor postures to the furniture on which they sit – and like children, adults would benefit also from sitting on the floor. Each time you join your child on the floor, monitor your own posture. Practising the tailor pose with your child can improve your flexibility, too.

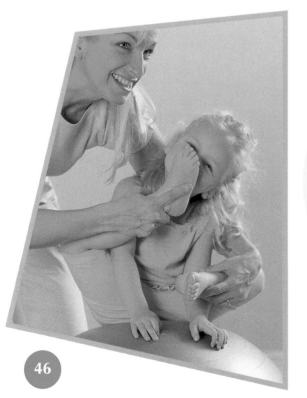

Practice Point

Remember to hold your child securely at all times when she is balanced on the exercise ball. If you would be more comfortable with some additional stability, you can deflate the ball slightly or position it close to a wall. For more information on using exercise balls, see page 25.

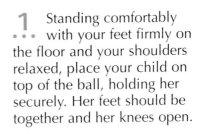

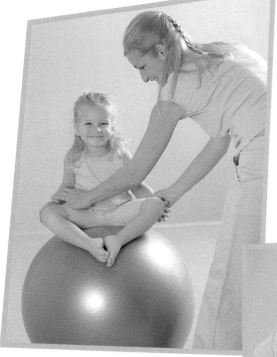

1 Standing comfortably with your feet firmly on the floor and your shoulders relaxed, place your child on top of the ball, holding her securely. Her feet should be together and her knees open.

2 Place your hands on her lower legs and rock her gently backwards and forwards on the ball.

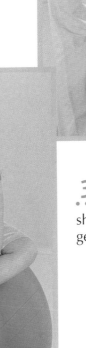

3 Now move your hands up to your child's shoulders and bounce her gently a few times.

47

Forward Bend

The hamstrings at the back of the thighs are postural muscles that help keep the body erect. While they have to be strong, they must also be supple so a child can bend forwards without placing undue strain upon her back and spine.

Flexible legs are of great advantage to posture and mobility, and also aid circulation. When relaxed, the postural muscles act like sponges, absorbing blood from the arteries, and when they contract, they squeeze blood back into the veins. This relaxation and contraction of the postural muscles enables them to act like pumps, assisting the circulation of blood back to the heart through the veins and against the force of gravity.

It can be difficult for children who have not been encouraged to maintain a wide range of movement as they grow stronger to achieve a forward bend. Many children find it hard to bend forwards with straight legs to touch the floor. If the hamstring muscles can relax freely, you should be able to bend from the waist, with your knees straight, and place the palms of your hands on the floor. Try to keep this exercise light and fun.

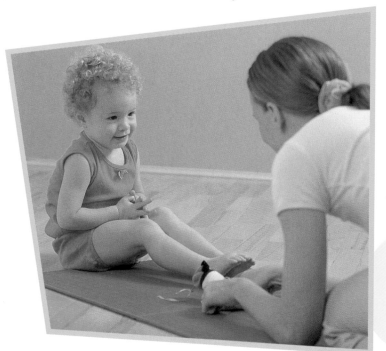

Fun and games
Allow your child to take a break between exercises, to play with one of her favourite toys, or just to run around freely.

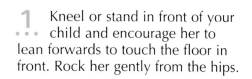

1 Kneel or stand in front of your child and encourage her to lean forwards to touch the floor in front. Rock her gently from the hips.

2 Still holding her at her hips, let her bend her knees and lower her head towards the floor, with her chin tucked in.

3 Still holding her from her hips, help her to roll forwards and up onto her hands, until her bottom lands on your knees. Repeat this 3 or 4 times, stopping if your child gets bored.

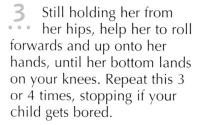

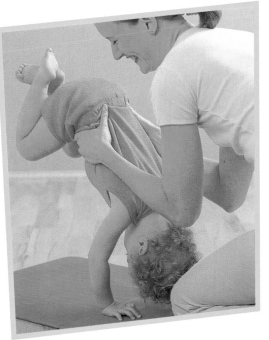

Alternatively

You can try this exercise using an exercise ball for variation. Stand comfortably and hold your child's hands and forearms as she sits on the ball facing you with straight legs pointing towards you.

Help her to lean forwards by slowly letting the ball roll backwards. Now roll her forwards again, repeating this 2 or 3 times.

Bringing your child onto the top of the ball again, hold her upper body and bounce her gently 3 or 4 times or more, taking her chest towards her legs each time.

Side Splits

When jumping or dancing or trying to regain his balance during play, your child will often open his legs wide to the side to give himself a broader base. All upright structures, whether a boy or a building, depend upon their foundations – so when the legs are both strong and flexible and can open into a broad base, your child will feel secure.

Unlike the back or the shoulders, the hip joints hide their stiffness easily. Any tension will become apparent only when your child stretches open his legs sideways. If the adductors, or inside thigh muscles, tighten and the legs cannot open sideways easily, sitting in tailor pose (see page 42) becomes more difficult. This may result in your child adopting less healthy sitting positions. Side splits will help to maintain the condition of these essential muscles.

Add to the fun by engaging your child's imagination in your practice: your child can be a cowboy or cowgirl trying to maintain a firm seat upon a mischievous horse.

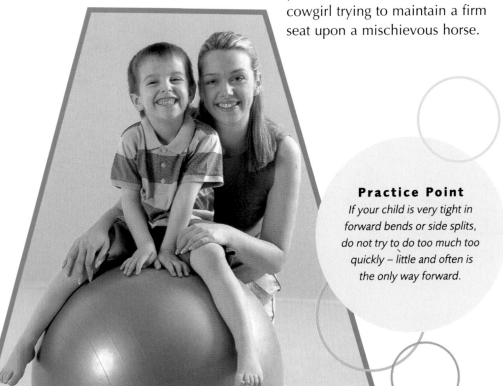

Practice Point

If your child is very tight in forward bends or side splits, do not try to do too much too quickly – little and often is the only way forward.

1   Standing comfortably in front of your child, hold him by his hands and forearms as he sits with his legs open astride the ball. Rock him sideways a few times to allow him to settle comfortably and begin to stretch his legs.

2   Still holding him firmly, encourage him to lean forwards by slowly rolling him backwards on the ball. Ask him to aim to remain firmly seated on the ball. Now roll him forwards again, then repeat 2 or 3 times or more, backwards and forwards.

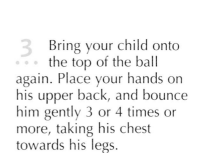

3   Bring your child onto the top of the ball again. Place your hands on his upper back, and bounce him gently 3 or 4 times or more, taking his chest towards his legs.

51

HEAD AND NECK FLEXIBILITY

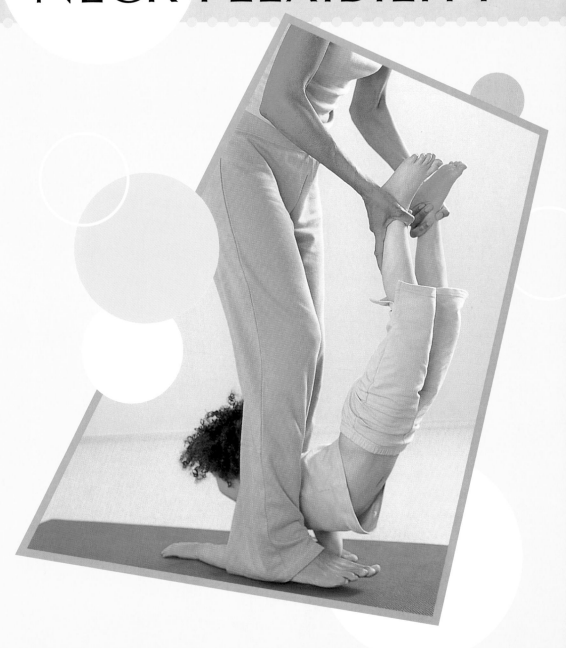

3

Key to a child's naturally vibrant posture
is the way she holds her head and neck.
With care and attention, the exercises in
this chapter will help to ensure a strong
and healthy physique for life.

Shoulderstand

Of all the yoga *asanas*, or postures, the shoulderstand is considered to be one of the most beneficial. It is said to regulate the blood pressure and to assist the venous return (the return circulation of blood to the heart). It also relieves any tension in the neck.

The neck is the most flexible part of the spine – it is the only section that allows full forward-bending. At the same time, the neck muscles and joints enable the head to rotate from shoulder to shoulder, to bend sideways to touch the ears to the shoulders, and to bend backwards as well as forwards.

The head, balanced upon the top of the spinal column, remains elevated and straight because of the equal pull from the muscles on all sides of the neck. Young children naturally hold their heads upright, without craning their necks forwards as many adults do. This healthy stretch will help your child maintain her good posture, because practising the shoulderstand encourages suppleness, strength and flexibility in the neck.

Practice Point

Your child should not turn or twist her head while she is in a shoulderstand. If she does, gently lower her to the ground without twisting her further.

1 With your child lying
on her back on the floor
facing you, hold her firmly from
the lower legs. Remember to
bend from the knees, keeping
your back straight, to prevent
any strain to your own back.

2 Slowly lift her legs
until she is resting on
the back of her shoulders.
Engage her by talking to
her and rocking her gently
from side to side before
lowering her down onto
her back again.

3 Once she is confident in
the shoulderstand, you can
encourage her to tuck her chin
towards her chest. This will
allow you to lift her legs higher,
enhancing the stretch.

55

Handstand

The handstand is an invigorating posture that allows extra blood and oxygen to reach the brain. It also increases the blood supply to the pituitary and pineal glands; the healthy functioning of these two glands support growth, health and vitality. In addition, this supported handstand can also lengthen and align the spine.

Some children at first may find it quite traumatic to be lifted upside down. One theory holds that this

1 Stand comfortably with your legs and feet slightly apart; your child should lie on her back on the floor facing you.

2 Hold your child firmly by her lower legs and gently lift her until the crown of her head is touching the floor, in a 'handstand'. You must support her entire weight. Hold for a few seconds before lowering her back down.

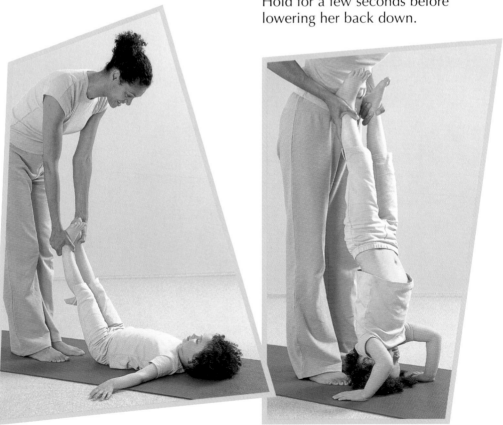

could be associated with birth; during most deliveries the baby descends head-first through the birth canal. If your child seems nervous or uncomfortable, start by lifting her from the floor gently, and a little at a time. Keep the exercise light and friendly, and if she shows signs of distress, stop and rock her gently. Repeat gradually until she is totally comfortable before you take it any further.

Alternatively
You can slide your child's body up your legs until she is supported by her hands.

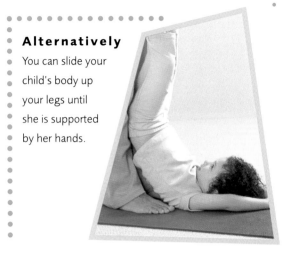

3 Once she is confident, you can encourage her to straighten her arms.

4 If her arms remain fully extended, lower her onto her tummy. If not, lower her onto her back. Repeat 2 or 3 times.

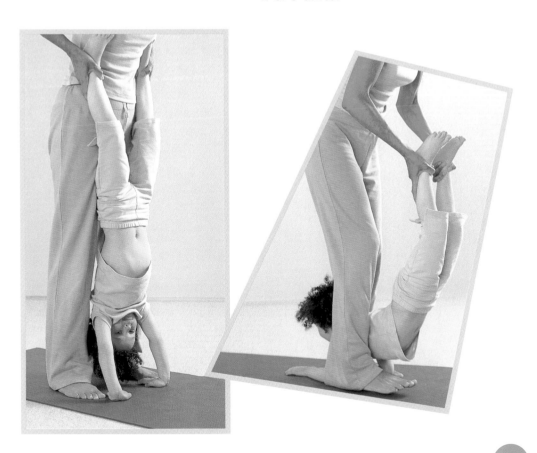

Handstand into Cobra

This exercise uses a ball to help support your child's weight, which means he may feel more confident, and it gives you the advantage of being able to keep the exercise a bit more playful. Bounce and rock your child gently, talking him through each step to make sure that he is completely relaxed before you proceed. Take your time and don't try to hurry your child.

As your child takes a little of his own weight in the handstand, he will be strengthening his arms and shoulders. Going from this position into the cobra will help to keep his shoulders flexible and also will stretch his chest and abdomen.

1 Standing comfortably with your legs and feet apart, hold your child from his hips and let him bend backwards over the ball.

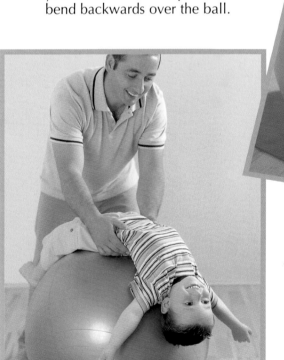

2 Slide your hands to a point just above his ankles and roll him back slowly until the crown of his head touches the floor. Repeat until he feels comfortable, then encourage your child to place his hands on the floor and push up as you bring him back onto the top of the ball. Repeat a few times.

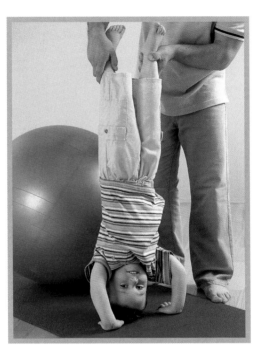

Practice Point

Remember to work on a soft surface to protect your child's face.

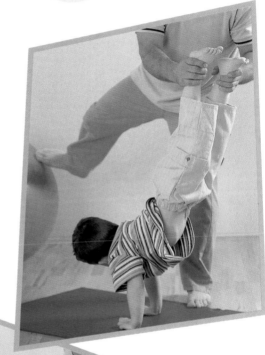

3 Move from behind the ball to stand to the side of your child, holding his legs firmly. Bring him carefully into a handstand position.

4 Encourage him to lift his head so that he can see the ball (*above right*). Then lower him onto the floor in a cobra position (*below right*). As you are doing this, you may need to move around or push the ball out of the way, but make sure that you do not release your grip on your child or twist him as you change your position.

BACKBENDS
AND BALANCING

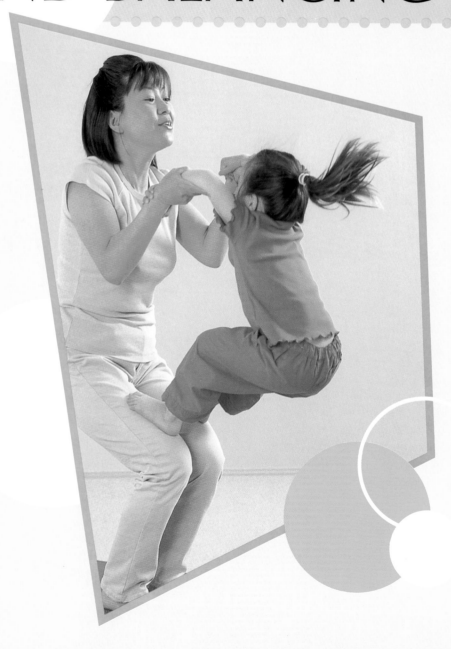

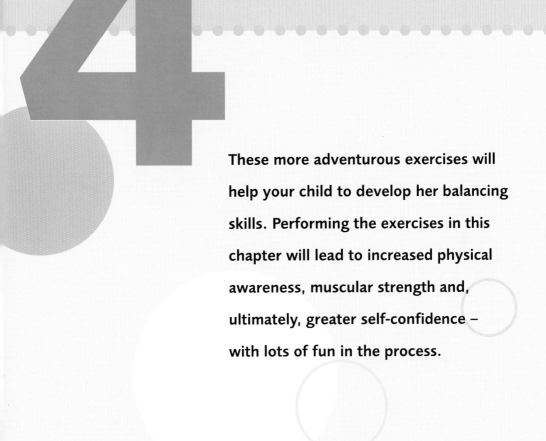

4

These more adventurous exercises will help your child to develop her balancing skills. Performing the exercises in this chapter will lead to increased physical awareness, muscular strength and, ultimately, greater self-confidence – with lots of fun in the process.

Leg Lifts

This exercise is one that many parents and children practise without any guidance or instruction. Because it comes naturally to most children, it rarely fails to delight, so it's a useful activity to bear in mind if your child needs a little encouragement to engage in some soft gymnastics.

The leg lifts on these pages are an ideal preparation for the more adventurous backbend that follows (see page 66). Do not try the more ambitious version until your child is totally comfortable being lifted as shown here – and until you, too, have the strength and confidence to support him with your legs and your forearms. Use this exercise also to work up to the more advanced backflip, which requires you to lift your child quite high with your legs, in order to catch him at the hips.

Practice Point

The position of your forearms is very important because the forearms are the primary supports for your child. If they brace him correctly, you will be able to control his movements once you have lifted him with your legs.

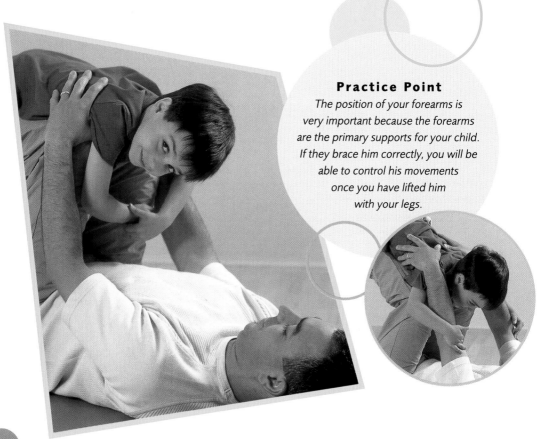

1 Lie comfortably on your back
with your head supported on
a cushion and your knees bent. Let
your child lie on your legs, with his
legs open over yours, his feet
towards your feet and his head
on your knees.

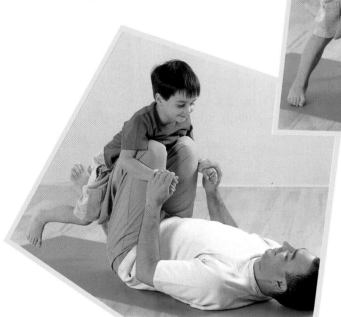

2 Relax and gently
rock him from
side to side.

3 Brace him with your
forearms against his
shoulders, before lifting
and lowering your legs.

Tip
*These exercises will help
you to strengthen your
own abdominal muscles.
To avoid back strain, make
sure your spine remains in
a neutral position. Do not
twist or arch your back.
Do not strain your neck.
Breathe in as you lift your
child up, using the breath
to ease the movement.*

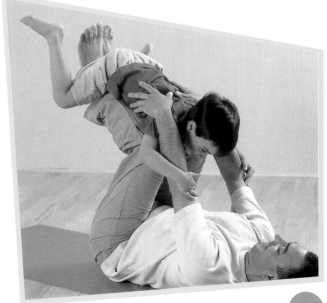

Topsy Turvy

This is a lovely stretch for your child. Suspended in the backbend, she can effortlessly open her chest and shoulders and stretch her abdomen. Your child will be so thrilled by the acrobatic nature of the exercise that she will want to repeat it over and over again.

Your firm support is crucial throughout this exercise. Do not attempt it until you have practised the Leg Lifts (see page 62) and feel confident with those. You will have to be able to lift your child quite high, bearing her weight largely with your legs, in order to transfer your grip to her hips before you raise her into the backbend.

It is important to keep your forearms braced on your child's shoulders as you lift her, to keep her from over-extending her spine. You must lift – not flip – your child into the backbend, supporting her throughout.

Practice Point

Take care of your back. Prevent strain by maintaining a neutral spine. If your back becomes uncomfortable, lower your child to the floor and relax for a few moments by lying on your side, with your knees bent.

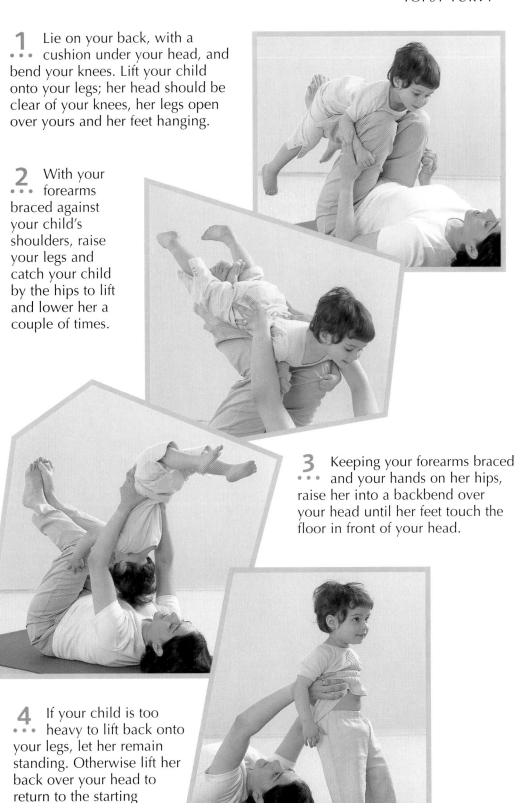

1 ••• Lie on your back, with a cushion under your head, and bend your knees. Lift your child onto your legs; her head should be clear of your knees, her legs open over yours and her feet hanging.

2 ••• With your forearms braced against your child's shoulders, raise your legs and catch your child by the hips to lift and lower her a couple of times.

3 ••• Keeping your forearms braced and your hands on her hips, raise her into a backbend over your head until her feet touch the floor in front of your head.

4 ••• If your child is too heavy to lift back onto your legs, let her remain standing. Otherwise lift her back over your head to return to the starting position on your legs.

Lift Offs

The way that you hold, touch and play with your child gives her a variety of messages. For a healthy child, a firm, confident touch will add to her sense of security. She learns not only that she is loved and wanted, but also that she is strong and resilient. Alternatively, if you treat your child as if she is made of glass, you are telling her that she is fragile, giving her a message of insecurity.

The exercise shown here is not about strength or flexibility. This time it is all about enhancing the relationship you have with your child. It is important that you remain attentive at all times, observing your child's reactions and responding to them affirmatively. If your child appears upset or startled by what you are doing, stop and leave it for a while – you may need to wait only a few moments, or you may need to wait a few days. The next time you try an exercise, proceed more slowly, singing or talking to offer reassurance and love.

Practice Point

This is an exercise to do only with very small children. Be aware of your own comfort level – do not strain your back or shoulders as you lift your child.

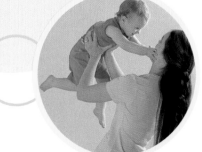

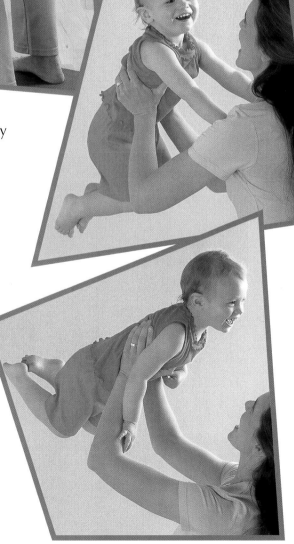

Tip

Each time you prepare to lift your child, offer a verbal clue – 'Ready, steady, go' or 'One, two, three' or the like – to let her know something is about to occur. This will help her to learn to associate these words with something special taking place.

1   Hold your child firmly around the chest, under her arms.

2   'Ready, steady, go', and lift her until you are face to face. Repeat a few times, as long as you are both enjoying yourselves.

3   'Ready, steady, go', and lift your child above your head. Again, repeat a few times.

Side Stretch and Swing

Like many of the soft gymnastics exercises in this book, this side stretch has multiple benefits. It helps to open the chest and shoulders, and it will also help to strengthen your child's arms and legs. Finally, it will stretch the sides of his chest, making his rib cage more flexible and his breathing more relaxed.

Take your time as you get started with this stretch, offering lots of reassurance at the outset. While most youngsters enjoy being

swung like this, they may be a little apprehensive at first. Soon, any nerves will probably give way to laughter.

However, even with loving preparation, some children may not enjoy being lifted in this way. If that is the case with your child, he will benefit from side stretches using the ball variation (see page 70).

Practice Point
Because your child's wrists and ankles are not yet fully formed, make sure you hold him from the forearm and lower leg. Also because the hip is a larger, stronger joint than the shoulder, it is best to take more of his weight through the leg.

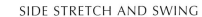

1 Keeping your legs apart for stability, bend from your knees and take hold of your child's left forearm and left lower leg.

2 Raise him slightly off the floor, allowing his right side to continue to rest on the floor and taking more of his weight through his leg than his arm. Lower, then repeat, for as long as you both are comfortable.

3 This time, lift your child off the floor and swing him gently from side to side, still taking more of his weight through his leg than his arm. His right arm may sweep lightly along the floor. To avoid any strain on your back, you can keep your knees bent and your shoulders relaxed. Lower, then repeat on the other side.

69

Side Stretch with Ball

Side stretching may be easier if you use an exercise ball, because the ball will support your child's weight, helping him to develop confidence in the action. Once he feels secure, then you can lift him up and off the ball, as in the previous exercise, to enhance the stretch. You may have to kick the ball lightly out of your way once you have lifted him off – pay attention to your own balance as you do so.

As with any exercise, it is important to wait until your child is totally secure and confident in the basic position before you attempt the more advanced variation suggested in step 3. Some children may not enjoy being lifted in this way, so pay close attention to your youngster's responses. At the first sign of apprehension, bounce or rock him lightly on the ball, and do not try to take the exercise further. Instead, repeat the stages with which he feels comfortable, in order to restore his confidence.

1 Stand securely with your legs and feet apart, your knees slightly bent, and let your child lie back over the ball. Hold him by his left forearm and left lower leg.

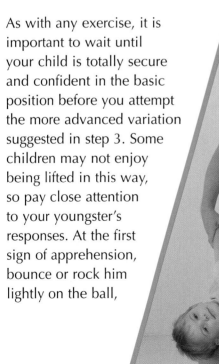

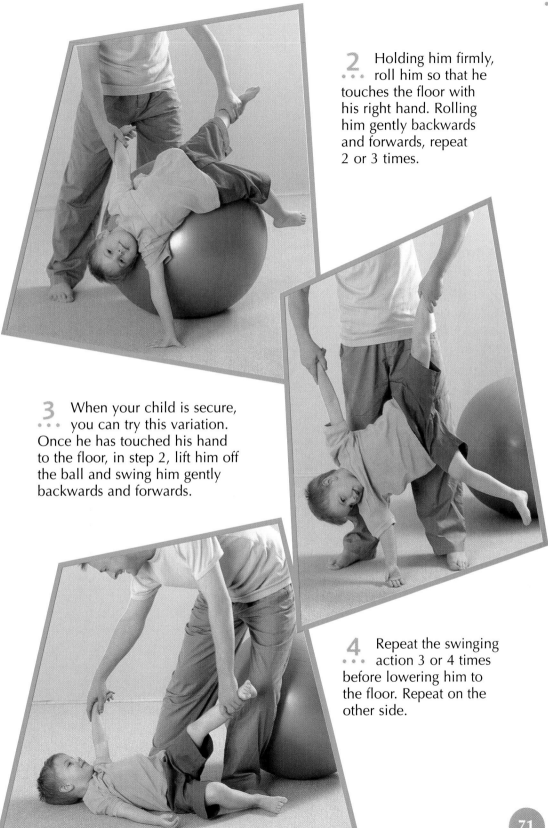

2 Holding him firmly, roll him so that he touches the floor with his right hand. Rolling him gently backwards and forwards, repeat 2 or 3 times.

3 When your child is secure, you can try this variation. Once he has touched his hand to the floor, in step 2, lift him off the ball and swing him gently backwards and forwards.

4 Repeat the swinging action 3 or 4 times before lowering him to the floor. Repeat on the other side.

71

Lookout

Most children love a hint of danger when they know they are in safe hands. They enjoy being thrown up in the air, caught, swung and balanced when they know they are supported by a loving, strong partner. This kind of play encourages a child's confidence.

When balancing, flexibility is all-important. If your child's ankles are supple, they will bend easily, allowing his body to remain upright while his feet twist to secure balance. If his ankles are inflexible, his whole body is thrown off balance when his feet twist. Lookout is an elementary exercise in balancing, providing a relatively safe introduction to this art. As your child climbs atop your legs, like a sailor ascending the mast of a ship, he will further strengthen and stabilise his legs and encourage flexibility in his feet and ankles.

As with all balances, even the most simple, there is a risk of falling. To be on the safe side, surround yourself with cushions and work on a soft, non-slip surface. Ensure that the position of your legs is secure, so that they will not buckle or twist when your child stands on them.

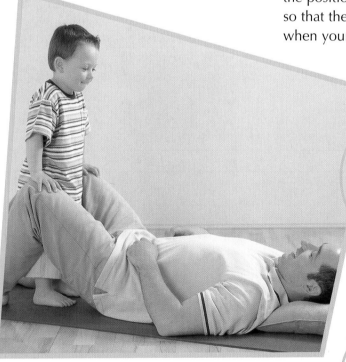

Practice Point

Make sure that your clothing is tight across your knees, so that it does not slide when your child stands on them. It is best for your child to have bare feet, so he can grip with his toes.

1 Lie on the floor on your back with your knees bent and a pillow under your head. Hold your child by his hands and forearms.

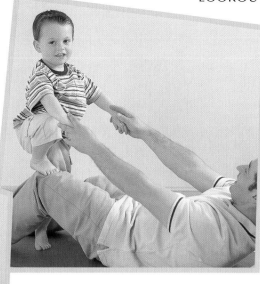

2 Holding your child firmly and keeping your knees pressed together, help him to climb up onto your knees.

3 Support and steady him with your hands, keeping his knees pressed together for stability. Only when you are both absolutely comfortable, release one hand at a time so your child balances, even just momentarily.

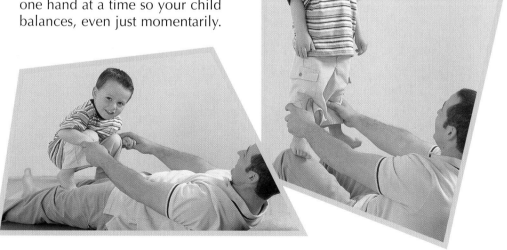

4 Take his hands again to help him return to the ground. You can slowly straighten your legs to lower him. Otherwise, he can step down carefully.

Moving Mountain

We are aware of our physical selves through a little-known sense called proprioception. Sense receptors, known as proprioceptors, are situated in the non-hearing part of the inner ear, as well as in the muscles, tendons and joints. They are stimulated by muscular activity, the movement of the joints and the positioning of the body in space, and they operate like little spirit levels, helping us to maintain our balance.

Proprioception is more developed in a flexible, agile body. Games and exercises that involve balance, such as this one, also stimulate this sense, helping it to develop. As this sense grows keener through practice, balancing becomes easier, and a high sense of physical awareness develops.

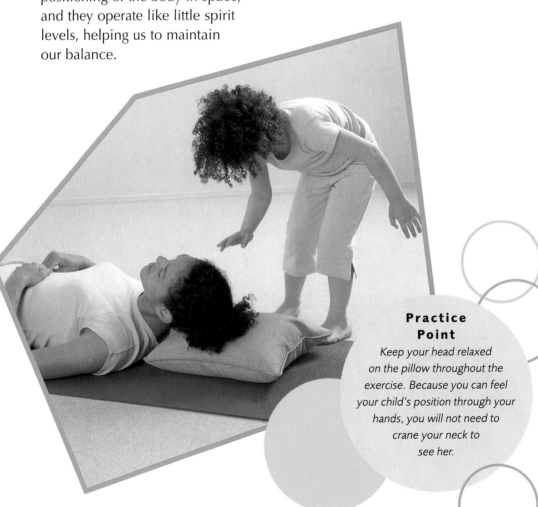

Practice Point

Keep your head relaxed on the pillow throughout the exercise. Because you can feel your child's position through your hands, you will not need to crane your neck to see her.

1 Lie on the floor with your head
••• on a pillow, your legs raised with
your knees bent, and your child sitting
astride your legs.

2 Support her under the soles of
••• her feet, keeping your elbows on
the floor and bracing your forearms
on your thighs for stability if necessary.

3 Slowly bearing more of
••• your child's weight on your
hands, straighten your legs, as she
leans against them for support,
perhaps holding them for security.

4 Once you both are steady,
••• she can balance on her
own. Keep your own legs
strong for support and security.

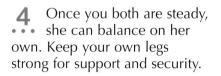

Walking on Your Shoulders

Many of the activities that children enjoy – climbing and balancing on available surfaces when young, delighting in cycling and skating when older – rely on their sense of balance. At the same time, these activities help to improve a youngster's balancing skills.

Balance games such as this one encourage both strength and coordination in the postural muscles and the muscles that support the spine.

Start gradually, with your child climbing only a small distance up your body. As he becomes more confident, he will want to climb higher and higher. Talk to your child throughout, reminding him to grip with his toes and to take his time, ascending one step at a time and placing his feet carefully, just as expert mountain climbers do. For a final challenge, see how long he can balance comfortably atop your shoulders as you support him lightly with your hands.

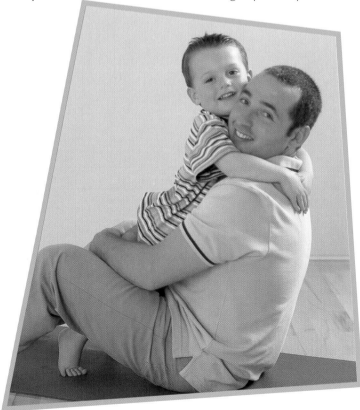

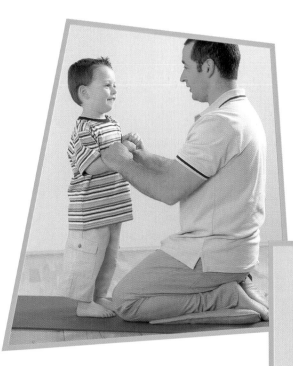

1 Begin by sitting on your feet on a cushion, with your child standing facing you. Hold him firmly by his hands and forearms.

2 As you lean back a little, let your child 'walk up' onto your shoulders. As he climbs, you must maintain a straight back and keep your abdomen firm.

4 Hold his hands against his hips as he balances atop your shoulders. After a few moments, help him to return gently to the floor, holding him securely.

3 If he is enjoying his ascent, let your child continue to climb up gradually until he finally reaches your shoulders.

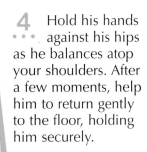

On Your Shoulders Stand

This exercise relies on trust and communication between you and your child. Not only will you have to maintain your own balance to provide a secure base for him, but you will also have to rely on your instincts, sensing when he is truly balanced before you begin to let go of one leg at a time. This kind of closeness and connection can only be nurtured through practice – it cannot be demanded.

1 Sit comfortably on your feet, on a cushion if you prefer, with your child standing facing you.

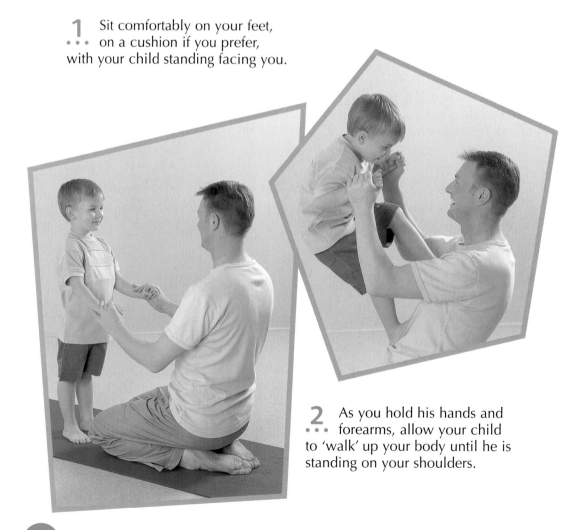

2 As you hold his hands and forearms, allow your child to 'walk' up your body until he is standing on your shoulders.

As a preliminary exercise, encourage your child to practise balancing on one leg. Once you see he can do this with both legs, you will know that he is ready to try the following balance.

As you work together, remember to keep your own back straight. Talk to your child, reassuring him and reminding him to take his time and relax.

Practice Point

It is easier to balance if you choose one fixed point to look at throughout the balance. Fix on something that is eye-level or higher, rather than looking down. Suggest a focal point to your child before he climbs up to your shoulders.

3 Carefully transfer your hold to his hips and legs.

4 When you are both in equilibrium, release one hand at a time, keeping your hands close for safety and a feeling of security. Enjoy the feeling of balance for a few moments.

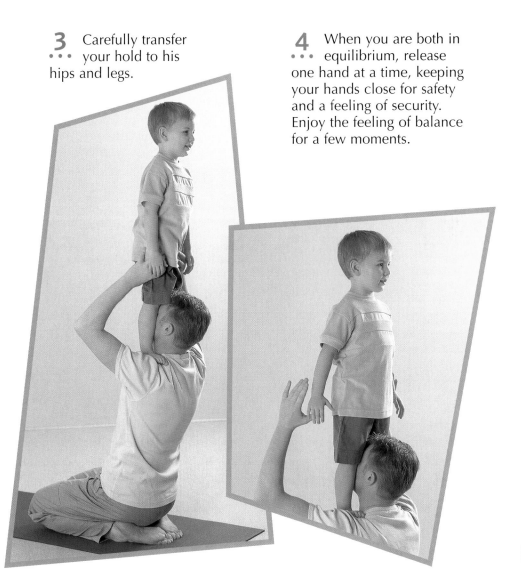

Shoulder Roll

Life is dynamic; life is movement. From birth onwards, your child's life force is continually expressed through the variety of her actions and positions.

Your child's innate love of movement is a source of joy and should be fostered. While there is a time for calm and gentle stretches, there must also be time for acrobatic and adventurous exercises such as the one shown here. Although it seems complicated, you will find that as you work together, the moves will fall naturally into place. Enjoy yourselves as you work together, and you can both have fun.

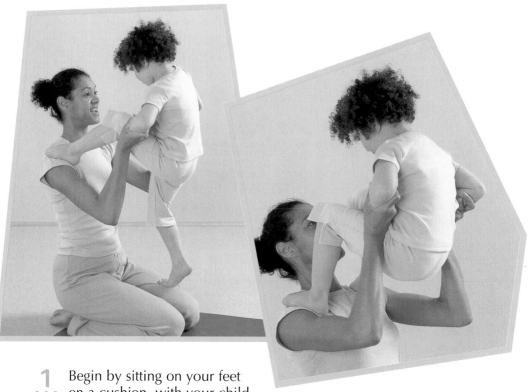

1 Begin by sitting on your feet on a cushion, with your child facing you. Holding her by the forearms, steady her as she walks up your body until she reaches your shoulders. Keep your own back straight as she climbs.

2 As your child bends her knees, getting down close to your body, kneel up to give her the momentum for her to roll backwards towards the floor.

Tip
*Younger children
may need more support,
perhaps rolling into your
lap or into a sitting position
on the floor.*

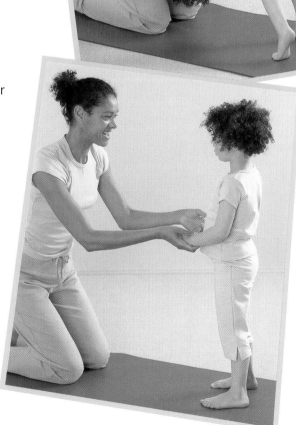

3 Keep your child
supported at all
times as she rolls
backwards, holding her
by the hips or by the
arms (*above left*), but
not by the hands or
wrists. This way you
will be able to control
her speed. Older
children will be able
to roll onto the floor,
ending in a standing
position (*below right*).

Backflip

Once your child is used to a backward roll, you can try taking this one step further, into a backflip. Although this may look complicated, youngsters take to the movements naturally. However, you should still proceed carefully. Make sure you hold your child by the hands and forearms because her wrists are not yet fully developed. Keep reminding your child to tuck in her chin as she flips backwards. This is useful advice for many activities, since there is less risk of injury to the neck if the chin remains tucked in.

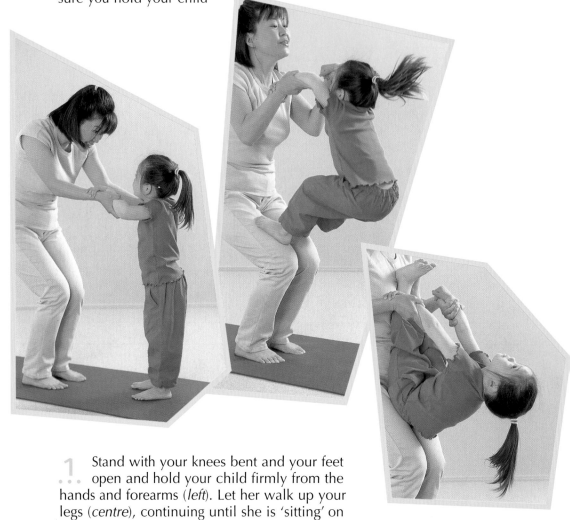

1. Stand with your knees bent and your feet open and hold your child firmly from the hands and forearms (*left*). Let her walk up your legs (*centre*), continuing until she is 'sitting' on your tummy (*right*).

Keep your feet open for stability and your knees bent, both to assist your child and to protect your lower back.

Once you and your child have mastered this flip, be prepared – your child will try to engage you in this game any time and any place, just for the sheer pleasure of it. She will also delight in showing off to her friends.

Tips

This is quite an advanced exercise and should only be attempted when you are both confident in your abilities. Some children take time before they enjoy being turned upside down. For them it is particularly important to start slowly and work up to this flip. Prepare by performing simple forward rolls on the floor; follow these with the Shoulder Roll (see page 80). Also, place lots of soft pillows or mats on the floor to cushion any falls.

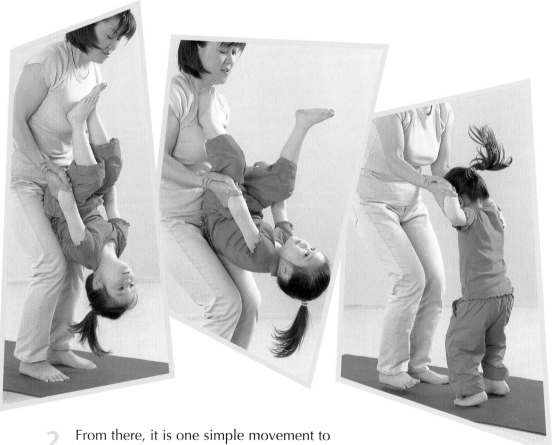

2 From there, it is one simple movement to flip around. Keep your own knees bent as she starts to bend her knees (*left*). You can help the flip to develop by pushing gently with your hips (*centre*) so that she ends up standing back on the floor (*right*).

ROLE-PLAYING EXERCISES

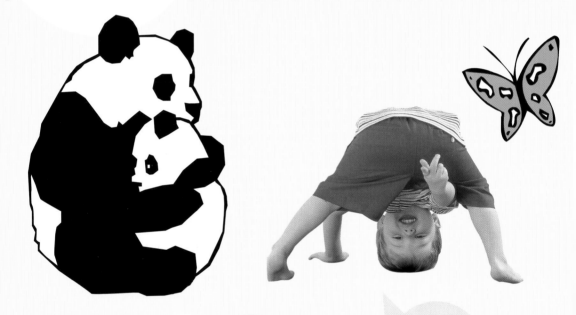

'Hey, Angie, look, I'm a gorilla!'

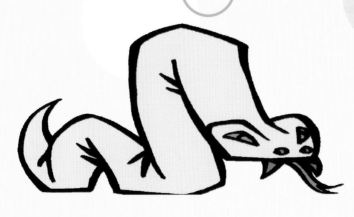

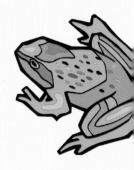

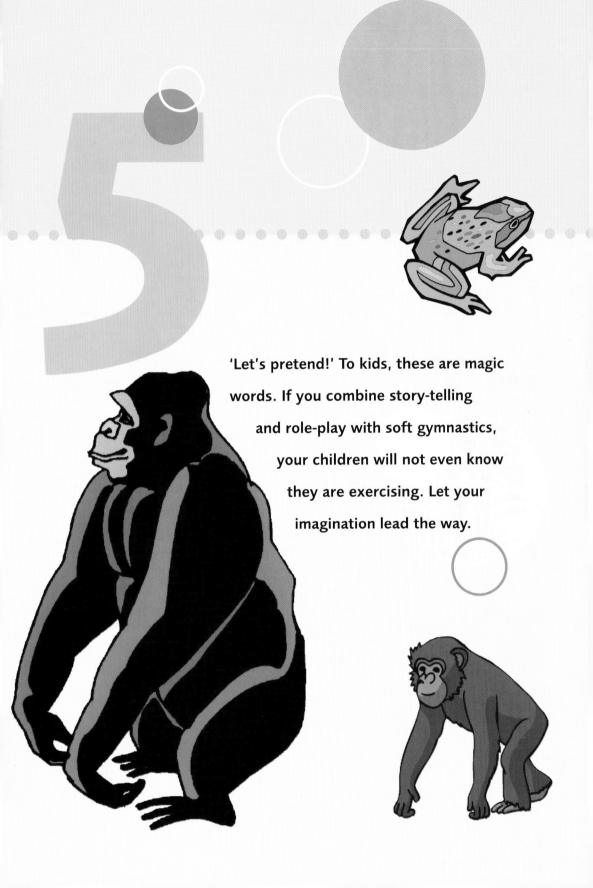

'Let's pretend!' To kids, these are magic words. If you combine story-telling and role-play with soft gymnastics, your children will not even know they are exercising. Let your imagination lead the way.

A Trip to the Zoo

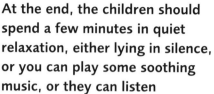

Children love stories and role-play games, so one way to encourage them to practise soft gymnastics is to incorporate several stretches into an engaging story. In fact, kids will have so much fun acting out the story that they will not even notice they are exercising. Here, a number of key exercises are woven into a story about a group of children taking a class trip to the zoo.

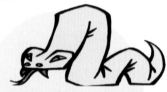

You can use this interactive story either with one child or with a group. As you read the story, there are cues for the kids to emulate certain behaviour.

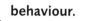

At the end, the children should spend a few minutes in quiet relaxation, either lying in silence, or you can play some soothing music, or they can listen as you talk to them gently – maybe about the feeling of warm sunshine on their faces and the other pleasing sensations of summertime.

Once you are familiar with the theme, feel free to personalise the story as you like. Change the name of the school to that of your child's school or play group, for example. Alternatively, you can use the story as a game at your child's birthday party, and change the school trip into a birthday treat, replacing the names with those of the guests.

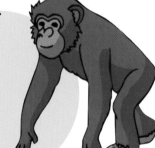

The children from Larkshill Primary School are very excited. Mr. Dawkins is taking them on a day's outing to visit the zoo. At the zoo, their teacher gathers all the children together. **'You must promise to behave,'** says Mr. Dawkins, **'and stop whatever you are doing when I ask you to.'** **'I will,'** says Angie. **'I can be as still as a tree.'**

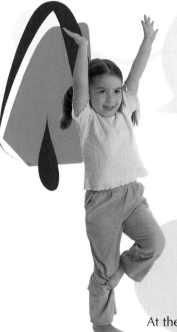

**'I will.
I can be as still
as a tree.'**

1 Angie stands silently. She raises one leg, placing that foot on her other leg for support.

2 She balances for a few moments, feeling as steady as an oak tree.

3 If she is confident of her balance, she raises her hands above her head, like the branches of a tree.

'Look, I can stand on my other leg as well,' says Angie, as she switches legs. With that, all the children in the class start to copy Angie.

Can you stand on one leg like a tree?

At the zoo the children go straight to the reptile house. They see a giant Indian snake. **'He's enormous,'** says Harry. The children look at the snake through the glass. Suddenly, the snake lifts its head, raises itself from the ground and lets out a loud hiss. **'He's talking to me,'** says Harry excitedly. **'I'll talk to him back.'**

1 Harry lies on the ground on his stomach, with his arms stretched out in front of him.

2 He lifts himself up onto his elbows, gently arching his back, raising his upper body.

3 He straightens his arms and, lifting his head and chest, he lets out a loud **'Hissssss'**. The snake hisses back, and Harry hisses back even louder.

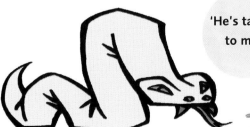

**'He's talking
to me.'**

Can you be a snake?

'**Look,**' squeals Mark suddenly, '**Over here! Come over here and look at this.**' The children hurry over to where Mark is standing, and there in front of him sits an enormous frog. '**Ribbett, ribbett,**' says the frog. '**Ribbett, ribbett, ribbett, ribbett.**' The children press their noses against the glass in their excitement, and as they do, the frog takes a giant leap into the air and disappears behind a rock.

'**I can jump farther than you.**'

'**That was a great jump** ' says Mark. '**I bet you couldn't jump like that,**' says Jane. '**Not like that? I bet I could,**' says Mark. '**I bet I could.**'

1 Mark drops down onto all fours, and spreads his knees and feet apart.

2 Raising himself up on his feet, he walks his hands back until his elbows are between his knees.

3 He then takes a great froggy leap forwards.

'**I can get my knees wider than yours,**' says Jane. '**I can jump farther than you,**' says Mark. Soon the whole class is jumping around like frogs.

Can you be a frog?

'**Come on, children,**' calls Mr. Dawkins. '**We have lots to see. All together now, line up and follow me.**' Mr. Dawkins leads the way, and soon the children arrive at a large open-air enclosure. It is full of trees and ropes and different kinds of swings. Over the top of the enclosure is a large sign. It reads GORILLAS. '**Hey, it's the Monkey House,**' says Peter. '**No it's not,**' says James. '**Gorillas are different from monkeys.**' '**Look,**' says Peter, '**Look at him, he's eating a banana.**'

'**I can get my knees wider than yours.**'

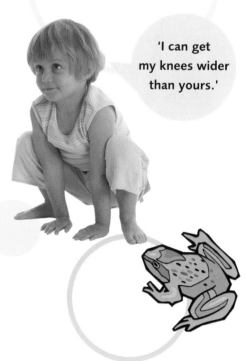

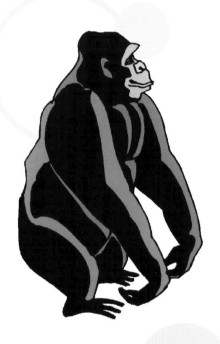

A large gorilla sits near the children, peeling a banana. The children watch, fascinated, as he eats the banana. Then he stands up, turning his back on the kids. **'Oh,'** says Angie. **'I think he's going to go away.'**

As if he'd heard what Angie said, the gorilla bends down and stares through his legs at the children. Then, leaning forwards, he rolls onto his back and stands up again. He turns to face the children, beating his chest with his hands. **'Wow,'** says Peter, **'That was great!'**

1 Bending his knees, Peter leans forwards and calls out, **'Hey, Angie, look, I'm a gorilla!'**

2 Peter straightens his knees and looks through his legs, laughing.

3 Then Jason joins in. Bending his knees, he tucks in his chin and rolls himself into a ball, before leaning forwards and doing a forward roll so that he ends up on his back.

4 Then Jason stands up, beating his chest with his hands. **'Hey, Peter, I'm a gorilla too.'**

'Hey, Angie, look, I'm a gorilla!'

'Hey, Peter, I'm a gorilla too.'

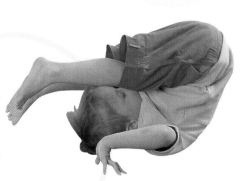

Can you be a gorilla?

'**Now, do keep up, children,**' says Mr. Dawkins. '**We're off to the insect house.**' The insect house is warm, and the children are entranced by the giant centipedes, spiders and enormous cockroaches. '**I'd like one of those,**' says Freddie, pointing to a large stick insect. '**I could frighten my mum with that,**' he adds, grinning.

'**Don't be mean,**' says Jane. '**Oh, look,**' she says, pointing to a large, brightly coloured butterfly. '**I'd love one of these.**' The children gaze at the big, beautiful butterfly and watch as she opens and closes her wings, stretching them until at last she flies up into the air and lands on a large fern leaf. '**I'd love to be a butterfly,**' says Angie, '**and then I could fly wherever I wished.**'

'**Look, I'm a butterfly.**'

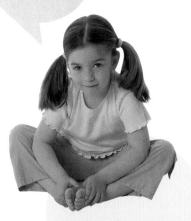

1 Angie sits down with her feet together and her knees open.

2 She takes hold of her feet with her hands.

3 Straightening her back, she pulls on her feet and opens her knees even wider, lowering them towards the floor. Then she gently flutters her knees up and down.

'**Look,**' she says, '**I'm a butterfly.**' Jane claps her hands with glee.

Can you be a butterfly?

'**Come along, come along,**' calls Mr. Dawkins. '**There's something special that I want you to see.**' The children follow excitedly and come to another enclosure with a forest of green bamboo. '**I can't see anything,**' says Tom.

'**I can,**' says Harry. '**Look over there!**' Harry points at a large black and white panda bear. '**Isn't he beautiful?**' he asks. '**It's not a he, it's a she,**' says Johnny. '**Look.**'

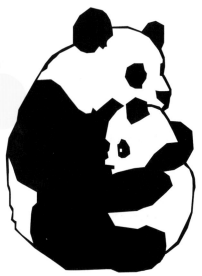

There, sitting by the side of the big panda bear, is a baby bear. He sits with one leg open and one leg closed. Then he opens both his legs, and, leaning forwards to stretch his back, he touches his toes. Then he sits up and rubs his head.

'**Ahhhhhh,**' say the children. '**Isn't he cute?**' '**Like me?**' asks Johnny. '**Am I cute too?**' The children turn to see Johnny.

'Like me?'
'Am I cute too?'

1 Johnny is sitting with one leg straight and one leg bent.

2 He straightens both his legs.

3 Then he leans forwards and touches his toes. All the children laugh.

Can you be a panda bear?

'**Follow me,**' says Mr. Dawkins. '**This way, and do keep together.**' The children follow their teacher until he stops in front of a group of chimpanzees. The baby chimps are chasing each other in circles. In the middle of the group sits a large, lazy, male chimpanzee. He is sitting between his feet. Then he leans back, placing his hands on his feet, and pushes his chest forwards. Resting back with his palms on the floor, he lets out a large sigh.

1 Like the chimpanzee, Jane is sitting between her feet.

2 Placing her hands onto her feet, she leans back and pushes out her chest.

3 Then she rests back with her palms flat on the floor, making a big sigh.

The big chimpanzee is watching Jane. He starts to jump up and down with excitement. All the children laugh.

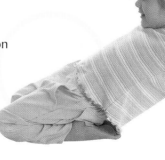

Can you be a chimpanzee?

Some noisy barking catches the children's attention. In the middle of a nearby patch of grass, a large dog is playing with a ball. A little boy is running after the dog, trying to get the ball back. The boy's parents are sitting on the grass having a picnic, and are laughing at the dog's antics. **'Hey, come on, Toby, give it back,'** says the little boy, as he tries to retrieve his ball. The dog takes no notice, and, holding the ball firmly in his mouth, he runs around and around the boy, teasing him.

The dog drops the ball and leans down on his front legs. He leans forwards and then stretches his chest, arching his back as he straightens his legs. The boy playfully imitates the dog.

1 He squats down in front of his dog.

2 Then he leans forwards, placing his hands in front of him.

3 He then presses backwards onto his heels, stretching his chest as he arches his back.

The dog looks on quietly, and all of a sudden, the boy jumps forwards and, snatching his ball, he runs off with his dog chasing after him. The children cheer.

Can you be a dog?

'All right,' says Mr. Dawkins. **'Who's ready for some lunch?'** The children are hungry and thirsty. It is a hot day and they have all brought sandwiches and fruit juice. They follow Mr. Dawkins to a large area of grass with the sign, **'Picnic Here'**, pinned to a tree in the middle.

Just as they are settling down, there is a lot of commotion as some of the zoo-keepers chase around several sheep who have escaped from the Petting Zoo. Freddie looks at his teacher. **'Mr. Dawkins,'** he says. **'Somebody forgot to close…'**

1 Angie stands facing forwards,
with her legs and feet wide apart.

2 She leans sideways, lowering her
left hand to her left ankle.

3 Then she raises her right hand high
into the air.

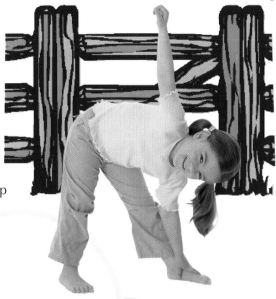

The children look puzzled. Angie stands up
and tries the same pose on the other side,
lowering her right hand to her right ankle.

'The gate!' shout all the children.
Mr. Dawkins laughs.

Can you be a gate?

The children have finished their lunch, and they are chattering loudly to each
other. **'All right,'** says their teacher. **'Let's have five minutes of quiet time before
we head off for home. I want you to be as quiet as shadows.'** The children lie
back on the grass, enjoying the warm sunshine. It has been an exciting day and
they are tired and happy.

1 They spread their arms and legs slightly
and close their eyes.

2 They feel themselves melt into
the soft grass.

Can you be as quiet as a shadow?

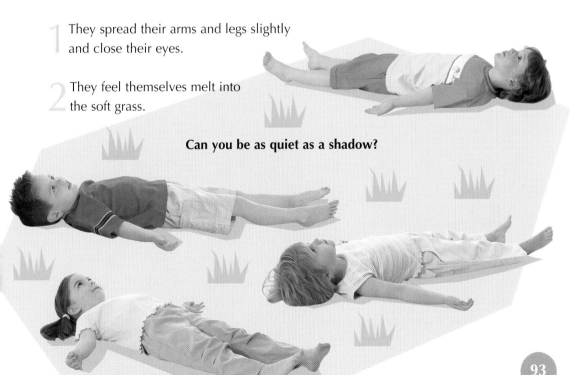

93

INDEX

ACKNOWLEDGEMENTS

The author would like to thank:

Becky Alexander, Michelle Bernard, Denise Brown, Amy Carroll, Frank Cawley, Stephanie Driver, Evie Loizides-Graham, Jules Selmes, David Yems and all the team at Carroll & Brown.

Heather and Emma at the Bubblegum agency for providing the models.

Models:

Alexander Antoniou, Ross Axton, Freddie Badham, Aliyah Butt, James Cundy, Joe Green, Maia Harris, Kameron Harvey-Smart, Olivia Haysman-Walker, Tabitha Hutchins, Georgie Mziu, Rio Otero, Oliver Peacock, Kyle Roullier, Ezria Rolfe, Harry Scott, Blayne Shiels, Charlie Taylor, Tess Turner, Charlotte Vaughan, Sunisa Visessombat, William Wilcocks

and a personal thanks to his son, Sauri Roche Walker, also for modelling.

Carroll & Brown would like to thank:

Production manager
Karol Davies

Production controller
Nigel Reed

Computer management
Paul Stradling

Make-up artist
Jessie Owen

Yoga mats by **Hugger Mugger Ltd**
12 Roseneath Place, Edinburgh, EH9 1JB
tel: 0131 221 9977
fax: 0131 221 9112
e-mail: info@huggermugger.co.uk
website: www.huggermugger.co.uk

Carpet by **Rainbow Carpets and Curtains**
413 Harrow Road, London, W9 3QJ
tel: 020 8964 8181